First Aid
Manual

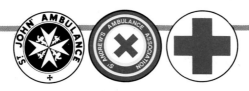

First Aid Manual

The Authorised Manual of
St. John Ambulance
St. Andrew's Ambulance Association
The British Red Cross Society

Dorling Kindersley · London

Fifth edition first published in Great Britain in 1987 by
Dorling Kindersley Limited, 9 Henrietta Street,
Covent Garden, London WC2E 8PS

First impression July 1987
Conjoint Societies 215,000 copies
Trade 43,000 copies
Second impression January 1988
Conjoint Societies 170,000 copies
Trade 30,000 copies
Reprint 1988
Trade 50,000 copies
Third impression January 1989
Conjoint Societies 185,000 copies
Fourth impression February 1990
Conjoint Societies 160,000 copies
Trade 30,000 copies
Fifth impression October 1990
Trade 40,000 copies
Sixth impression January 1991
Conjoint Societies 235,000 copies
Seventh impression June 1991
Eighth impression December 1991

British Library Cataloguing in Publication Data

First aid manual: the authorized manual of
St. John Ambulance, St. Andrew's Ambulance
Association and the British Red Cross
Society. — 5th ed.
1. First aid in illness and injury
I. St. John Ambulance Association and
Brigade   II. St. Andrew's Ambulance
Association   III. Red Cross. *British
Red Cross Society*
616.02'52   RC87

ISBN 0-86318-232-1
ISBN 0-86318-230-5 Pbk

FOREWORD

The fourth edition of the *First Aid Manual* of the Joint Voluntary Aid
Societies marked a departure from the classroom format of old manuals to
an easily understandable style with numerous step-by-step illustrations.
It became instantly popular with members of the Voluntary Aid Societies and
with the public.

Medicine is a science which is constantly developing and first aid needs to
keep abreast of recent advances. It is with this in mind that revision in this fifth
edition has become necessary, and certain chapters have been completely
rewritten. The sections on shock, unconsciousness, fractures and emergency
childbirth have been revised. Spinal injuries have received special attention to
ensure that the first aider is more aware of the possibility of spinal fractures in
specific accidents. The traditional advice "do not touch if you suspect spinal
fracture" remains sound for an ordinary first aider, but there are occasions
when other dangers force him to act before skilled help becomes available.

Fears expressed by first aiders concerning infection have given rise to a new
section on the principles of hygiene.

Throughout the book minor alterations have been made to keep in step with
international consensus concerning first aid procedures, and more explanation
has been given to clarify points which some had found confusing.

Conscious of the difficulties which alteration creates for hard-pressed
instructors, the editorial committee has allowed no change other than for
reasons of accuracy and clarity of expression.

St. John Ambulance
St. Andrew's Ambulance Association
The British Red Cross Society

CONTENTS

HOW TO USE THIS BOOK

The joint *First Aid Manual* contains all the information necessary for standard First Aid courses. The Voluntary Societies will, after careful assessment of the theoretical and practical knowledge of each candidate following a recognized course of instruction, award First Aid certificates.

The information in the *First Aid Manual* is divided into three main sections, each denoted by different page borders. The *Major First Aid Techniques*, those which are vital to save lives, are contained in one chapter at the front of the book; these pages are marked by a wide, red border. Here you will find the techniques for resuscitation and the control of bleeding.

The main section of the book contains chapters which deal generally with situations such as *Action at an Emergency* and *Procedure at Major Incidents*, and others which deal specifically with conditions relating to the major classifications such as *Asphyxia, Wounds & Bleeding, Circulatory Disorders* and *Unconsciousness*. In each case the condition is defined, a list of the possible symptoms and signs is given, and the recommended treatment is described. The treatments are all set out in simple step-by-step form and are accompanied by clear illustrations to make them easier to follow. It is also important to realize that all the symptoms and signs listed as part of any condition do not necessarily occur in the order given and may not all be present in every condition.

Towards the end of the book are two chapters – *Dressings & Bandages* and *Handling & Transport* – which contain information relevant to all conditions. These chapters are denoted by wide, grey borders.

As a general principle, information on the structure and function of parts of the body has been included in appropriate chapters in order to aid understanding of the treatment described. These sections are contained in yellow tinted boxes.

The chapter on *Emergency Childbirth* at the end of the book is included to provide the necessary information should the emergency arise without normal facilities being immediately available. This subject, however, does *not* form part of a Standard First Aid course and is therefore *not* required for any examination purposes.

NOTE

The *First Aid Manual* can be used as a guideline for treatment by the untrained. However, the life-saving techniques of Artificial Ventilation and External Chest Compression should *not* be used until you have received proper instruction from a qualified instructor.

THE PRINCIPLES & PRACTICE OF FIRST AID

First Aid is the first assistance or treatment given to a casualty for any injury or sudden illness before the arrival of an ambulance or qualified medical expert. It may involve improvising with facilities and materials available at the time.

THE AIMS OF FIRST AID

First Aid treatment is given to a casualty:
- To preserve life.
- To prevent the condition worsening.
- To promote recovery.

THE RESPONSIBILITY OF THE FIRST AIDER

Because of the frequency and serious nature of many accidents, the role of the First Aider is very important.

In the management of a casualty, your responsibility as a First Aider is to:
- Assess the situation without endangering your own life.
- Identify the disease or condition from which the casualty is suffering (diagnosis).
- Give immediate, appropriate and adequate treatment, bearing in mind that a casualty may have more than one injury and that some casualties will require more urgent attention than others.
- Arrange, without delay, for the disposal of a casualty to a doctor, hospital or home, according to the seriousness of the casualty's condition.

Your responsibility ends when the casualty is handed over to the care of a doctor, a nurse or other appropriate person. You should not leave the incident until you have made your report to whoever takes charge and have ascertained whether you could be of any further help.

DEFINITIONS

Medical aid indicates treatment by a doctor at a hospital or surgery or at the scene.
First Aider is the term which describes any person who has received a certificate from an authorized training body indicating that he or she is qualified to render First Aid. It was first used in 1894 by the Voluntary First Aid Organizations.

First Aid certificates issued by St. John Ambulance, St. Andrew's Ambulance Association and the British Red Cross Society are awarded to candidates who have attended a course of theoretical and practical work and who have passed a professionally supervised examination.

The certificate awarded is valid only for three years thus ensuring First Aiders are:
- Highly trained.
- Regularly examined.
- Kept up-to-date in knowledge and skill.

MAJOR FIRST AID TECHNIQUES

Skilled First Aiders can save lives by maintaining a casualty's vital needs. The ABC rule will help you identify these needs:

A An open *Airway*
B Adequate *Breathing*
C Sufficient *Circulation*.

For life to continue, a person must be able to take oxygen into the lungs. This will, in turn, be distributed throughout the body by the blood. While it is possible for some parts of the body to survive for a time without oxygen, certain organs are very quickly affected – vital nerve cells in the brain can die after only three minutes.

The three emergency situations where a casualty is especially at risk because of interference with vital needs are:

- Lack of breathing and/or heartbeat.
- Severe bleeding.
- A state of unconsciousness which, as it develops, is likely to interfere with the open airway and eventually breathing.

(The order may vary according to the particular situation.)

The techniques in this chapter are:

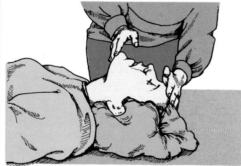

A AIRWAY *Opening the airway* to allow unobstructed passage of fresh air to the casualty's lungs.

The *Recovery Position* to help maintain an open airway so preventing the unconscious casualty becoming asphyxiated.

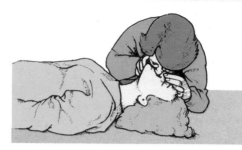

B BREATHING *Artificial Ventilation* to get air into the lungs of a casualty who has stopped breathing.

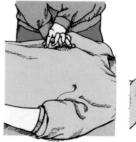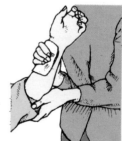

C CIRCULATION *External Chest Compression* to apply pressure on the chest and so pump blood through the arteries to the vital organs.

Controlling severe bleeding to prevent or minimize serious blood loss so that a casualty's circulation can be maintained.

A knowledge of how the body functions during respiration and circulation will help you apply these special techniques.

NOTE

It is important to practise these first aid techniques under trained supervision as no text book description is a substitute for practical knowledge and experience.

RESPIRATION

Oxygen is vital to support life. Breathing enables air to be taken into the lungs so that oxygen from the air can be transferred to the blood and circulated throughout the body, and allows carbon dioxide, a waste product, to be expelled.

When we breathe, air is drawn in at the nose or mouth and sucked down a main airway, the windpipe (trachea), through smaller passages (bronchi), and finally reaches air sacs (alveoli) in the lungs where an exchange of gases is made. Here, oxygen is picked up by the blood and carbon dioxide is given up by the blood to be breathed out.

Air is a mixture of gases: about 20 per cent of it is oxygen. Only some of this oxygen is used up, so that the air we breathe out contains 16 per cent oxygen in addition to a small amount of carbon dioxide. The amount of exhaled oxygen is thus adequate to resuscitate another person.

In the mouth and throat, food and air share the same passage. At the top of the main airway is the voice box (larynx) which not only serves as the organ of speech, but also acts to close off the air passages whenever you swallow, thus preventing the inhalation of food or drink. However, in an unconscious person, this protective mechanism works less well and becomes increasingly ineffective as unconsciousness deepens.

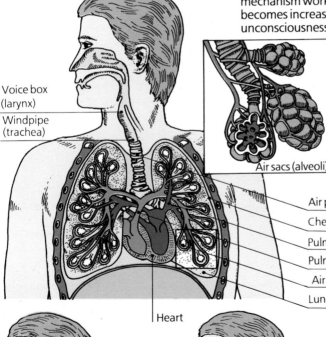

Respiratory system
On breathing in, air passes down the trachea, through the bronchi to the alveoli. Here, oxygen is picked up by the blood in exchange for carbon dioxide.

Voice box (larynx)

Windpipe (trachea)

Air sacs (alveoli)

Air passages

Chest cavity

Pulmonary vein

Pulmonary artery

Air sac (alveolus)

Lungs

Heart

Food

Epiglottis

Passage of air

Voice box (larynx)

Food

Oesophagus

Swallowing
To prevent food being inhaled, the epiglottis covers the entrance to the larynx, and food passes into the oesophagus.

How we breathe

Breathing consists of three phases: breathing-in (inspiration), breathing-out (expiration) and pause. When we breathe in, the chest muscles pull the ribs upwards causing the chest to expand in width and height. The diaphragm, a strong muscular partition which separates the chest cavity from the abdominal cavity, contracts and flattens increasing the chest's capacity from below. This combined action causes air to be sucked into the lungs so that the exchange of gases can take place. When breathing out, the diaphragm and the rib muscles relax and resume their position at rest. A short pause follows before the cycle starts again.

In normal respiration some residual air is left in the lungs so that some oxygen is always available to the circulating blood.

A respiratory centre in the brain determines the rate and depth of breathing: the average adult normally breathes 16–18 times per minute, whereas children and infants breathe 20–30 times per minute. This rate often increases during stress, exercise, injury or illness. The heart rate will increase accordingly to carry the extra oxygen around the body.

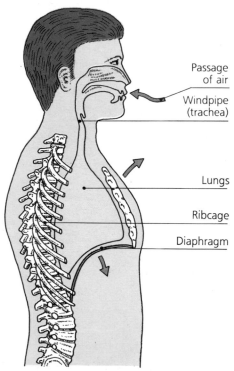

Passage of air

Windpipe (trachea)

Lungs

Ribcage

Diaphragm

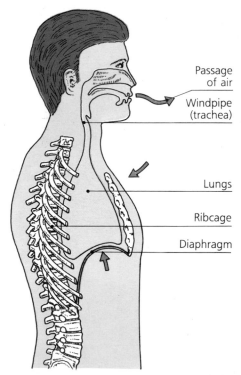

Passage of air

Windpipe (trachea)

Lungs

Ribcage

Diaphragm

Inhalation
As the diaphragm flattens and the ribcage moves upwards and outwards, the chest cavity is enlarged, reducing air pressure in the lungs. More air is then drawn into the lungs.

Exhalation
When the diaphragm and rib muscles relax, the ribcage moves downwards and inwards and the tissues of the lungs contract, thus forcing air out of the lungs.

How oxygen is circulated in the blood

Oxygen is carried around the body by the red cells in the blood (see p.84). Blood is circulated in a continuously repeated cycle by the contraction – relaxation movement of the heart. Each time the heart muscle (myocardium) contracts, blood is forced out of the pumping chambers of the heart; when the muscle relaxes, replacement blood pours into its collecting chambers. In the average adult at rest the heart "beats" 60–80 times per minute.

Deoxygenated blood flows back from the tissues into two main veins, and then into the right side of the heart. It is then forced out of the heart to the lungs where the exchange of gases takes place. The oxygenated blood returns to the left side of the heart and is then "pumped" out again into the main artery (aorta) from where it is distributed to all parts of the body (see *Blood & the Circulation*, p.26). Valves in the heart ensure that blood continues to flow in one direction.

The oxygenated red blood cells give the blood its bright red colour; blueness (cyanosis) arises when the blood is low in oxygen; pallor results from a reduction of blood in the skin. These colour changes are especially noticeable in the lips, earlobes and nail beds.

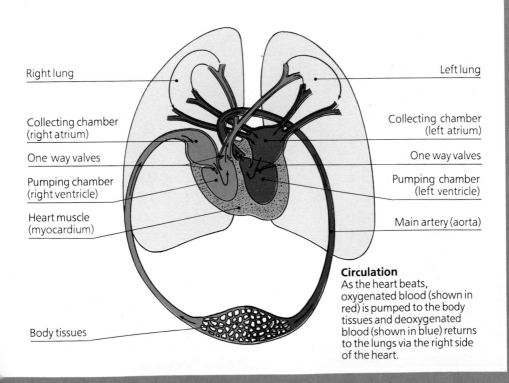

Right lung

Left lung

Collecting chamber (right atrium)

Collecting chamber (left atrium)

One way valves

One way valves

Pumping chamber (right ventricle)

Pumping chamber (left ventricle)

Heart muscle (myocardium)

Main artery (aorta)

Body tissues

Circulation
As the heart beats, oxygenated blood (shown in red) is pumped to the body tissues and deoxygenated blood (shown in blue) returns to the lungs via the right side of the heart.

RESUSCITATION

If a casualty is not breathing and if the heart is not beating, it is vital that you take over ventilation and circulation so that the flow of oxygen to the brain is maintained. Remember the ABC rule (see p.10). First, ensure an open **airway**; second, **breathe** for the casualty by inflating the lungs and oxygenating the blood (Artificial Ventilation); third, **circulate** the blood by compressing the chest (External Chest Compression).

The quick and efficient use of Artificial Ventilation, if necessary combined with External Chest Compression, should preserve the casualty's life until more skilled help is available. Resuscitation should be attempted even if you are in doubt about whether a casualty is capable of being revived. You should always continue until: spontaneous breathing and pulse are restored; another qualified person takes over; a doctor assumes responsibility for the casualty; or you are exhausted and unable to continue.

A OPENING THE AIRWAY

If a casualty is unconscious, the airway may be narrowed or blocked making breathing noisy or impossible. This occurs for several reasons: the head may tilt forward narrowing the air passage; muscular control in the throat will be lost, which may allow the tongue to sag back and block the air passage; and, because the reflexes are impaired, saliva or vomit may lie in the back of the throat blocking the airway. Any of these situations can lead to the death of the casualty so it is imperative that you establish a clear airway immediately.

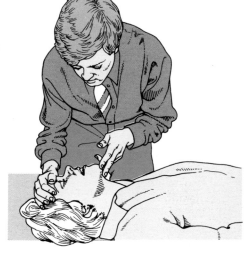

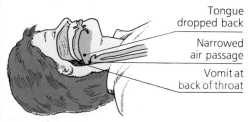

Tongue dropped back

Narrowed air passage

Vomit at back of throat

1 Kneel beside the casualty.

2 Lift her chin forwards with the index and middle fingers of one hand while pressing her forehead backwards with the heel of your other hand. Her jaw will lift her tongue forward, clear of the airway.

IF the casualty's breathing is or becomes noisy, her airway is obstructed. Open and clear her airway immediately.

NOTE
Once the airway is open, the casualty may begin breathing spontaneously. If she does begin breathing, place in the Recovery Position (see p.24). If she still does not breathe, begin Artificial Ventilation immediately (see p.18).

CHECKING BREATHING

In order to find out whether an unconscious casualty is breathing, after first opening the airway, look, listen and feel for any signs of respiration.

1 Continue holding the casualty's airway open (see left) and place your ear above her mouth and nose.

2 Look along her chest and abdomen. If she is breathing, you will hear and feel any breaths on the side of your face and see movement along her chest and abdomen.

CLEARING THE AIRWAY

Even when you have opened the casualty's airway, foreign matter such as vomit, loose teeth or dentures, or food may block the airway, thereby preventing the casualty from breathing. Any object that can be seen or felt should therefore be removed if possible.

1 Turn the casualty's head to the side, keeping it well back.

2 Hook your first two fingers and sweep round inside the mouth. But, *do not spend time searching for hidden obstructions and make sure that you do not push any object further down the throat.*

3 Check breathing again (see above).

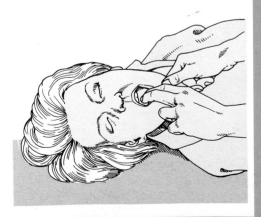

B BREATHING

The technique of breathing for a casualty is known as Artificial Ventilation. The most efficient method is to transfer air from your own lungs into the casualty's, by blowing into them through the mouth (Mouth-to-Mouth Ventilation). Sometimes, however, this is not possible in which case you may have to use a manual method (see p.216).

MOUTH-TO-MOUTH VENTILATION

The air we exhale contains about 16 per cent oxygen which is more than is needed to sustain life (see *Respiration*, p.11). In Mouth-to-Mouth Ventilation you blow air from your lungs into the casualty's mouth or nose (or mouth and nose together in a child) to fill the casualty's lungs. When you take your mouth away, the casualty will breathe out as the elastic chest wall resumes its shape at rest. Mouth-to-Mouth Ventilation enables you to watch the casualty's chest for movement, indicating that the lungs are being filled or that the casualty is breathing again naturally, and to observe changes in the casualty's colour (see p.21).

Mouth-to-Mouth Ventilation can be used by First Aiders of any age and in most circumstances. It is easiest to carry out if the casualty is lying on his or her back, but it should be started immediately – whatever position the casualty happens to be in. The first two inflations must be given slowly. The casualty may start breathing again at any stage but may need assistance until breathing settles down into a normal rate.

Mouth-to-Mouth Ventilation may not be suitable or possible in certain circumstances: if there are very serious facial injuries; if the casualty is pinned face downwards; or if there is evidence of corrosive substances around the mouth (see p.152).

For detailed instructions of how to give Mouth-to-Mouth Ventilation, see pp.18–19.

> **NOTE**
> Future references to Mouth-to-Mouth Ventilation include Mouth-to-Nose and Mouth-to-Mouth-and-Nose.

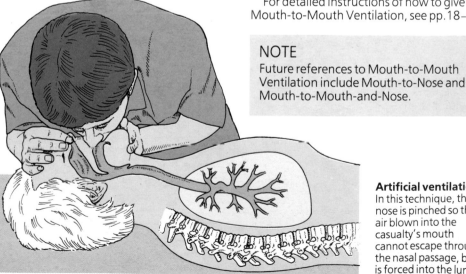

Artificial ventilation
In this technique, the nose is pinched so that air blown into the casualty's mouth cannot escape through the nasal passage, but is forced into the lungs.

C CIRCULATION

It is pointless continuing Artificial Ventilation if the casualty's heart is not beating, because the oxygenated blood will not be circulating. After the first two ventilations you must check carefully to see whether the heart is beating (see below). Always remember that while it is sometimes acceptable to assist breathing which is failing, the heart action is easily upset, so *never attempt External Chest Compression if the heart is beating, even faintly, and any pulse is felt.*

EXTERNAL CHEST COMPRESSION

Contractions can be simulated in a non-beating heart by compressing the chest. By pressing down on to the lower half of the breastbone you increase the pressure inside the chest thus driving blood out of the heart and into the arteries. When you release the pressure, the chest returns to its normal position and blood flows back along the veins and refills the heart as it expands.

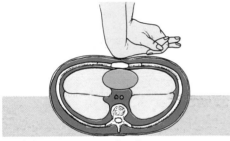

Applying pressure to the chest
This simulates contraction of the heart muscle causing blood to be pushed out of the heart.

External Chest Compression is *always* preceded, and accompanied, by Artificial Ventilation. To be effective, it must be carried out with the casualty lying on a firm surface. As soon as you feel a spontaneous pulse returning to the carotid artery stop External Chest Compression immediately, but carry on with Artificial Ventilation on its own, if it is necessary.

For detailed instructions on giving external chest compression, see pp.20–21.

CHECKING FOR CIRCULATION

Before commencing External Chest Compression it is very important that you establish that there is no circulation. Although the casualty may be blue around the lips (cyanosed) if the heart is not pumping blood to the surface, the only reliable way of establishing a lack of circulation is to check the pulse at the neck (carotid pulse). This pulse can be felt by placing your finger tips gently on the voice box and sliding them down into the hollow between the voice box and the adjoining muscle. (The pulse at the wrist is unreliable.) It must be checked again after the first minute and then every three minutes thereafter. It will only return spontaneously if the heart is beating.

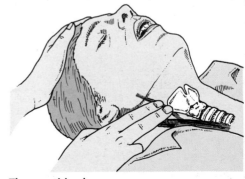

The carotid pulse
This is the wave of pressure which passes along the carotid artery as the heart beats.

MOUTH-TO-MOUTH VENTILATION

This is the preferred method of Artificial Ventilation in *all* cases where a casualty is not breathing (except for the few listed on p. 16). If the mouth cannot be used, satisfactory ventilation can be achieved through the nose (Mouth-to-Nose) or through the mouth and nose in small children and infants (Mouth-to-Mouth-and-Nose).

NOTE
Give the first two inflations as soon as possible; do not spend time looking for hidden obstructions.

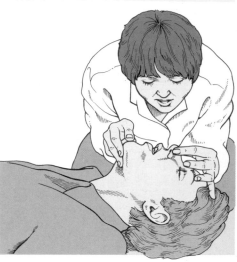

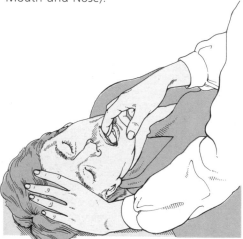

1 Remove any obvious obstructions over the face or constrictions around the neck. Open the airway (see p. 14) and remove any debris seen in the mouth and throat.

2 Open your mouth wide, take a deep breath, pinch the casualty's nostrils together with your fingers and seal your lips around his mouth.

MOUTH-TO-NOSE VENTILATION
If it is not possible to carry out Mouth-to-Mouth Ventilation, close the casualty's mouth with your thumb and seal your lips about his nose. Proceed as for Mouth-to-Mouth Ventilation (steps 3–5).

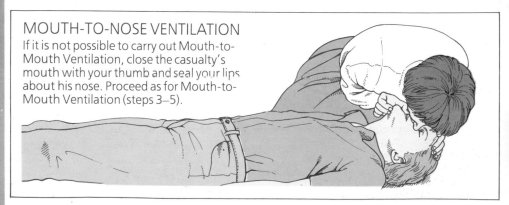

3 Blow into the casualty's lungs, looking along his chest, until you can see his chest rise to maximum expansion.

NOTE
If the casualty's chest fails to rise, first assume his airway is not fully open. Adjust the position of his head and jaw and try again. If there is still no ventilation, his airway may be blocked, and you will have to treat for *Choking* (see p.48).

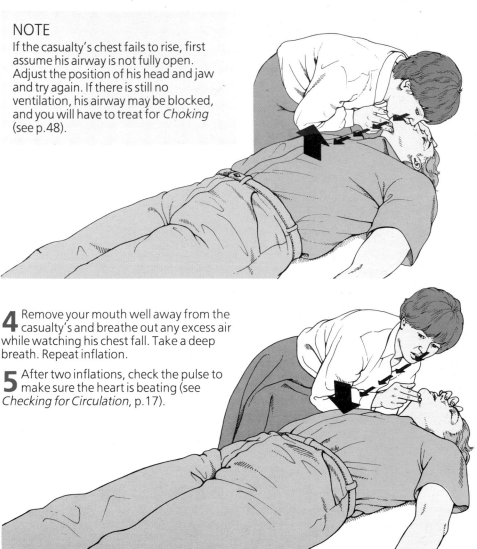

4 Remove your mouth well away from the casualty's and breathe out any excess air while watching his chest fall. Take a deep breath. Repeat inflation.

5 After two inflations, check the pulse to make sure the heart is beating (see *Checking for Circulation*, p.17).

IF the heart is beating and a pulse is felt, continue to give inflations at a rate of 12–16 times per minute until natural breathing is restored, assisting it when necessary and adjusting it to the casualty's breathing rate. When the casualty is breathing independently, place him in the Recovery Position (see p.24).

IF the heart is not beating you must perform External Chest Compression immediately (see overleaf).

EXTERNAL CHEST COMPRESSION

If Mouth-to-Mouth Ventilation by itself is unsuccessful and the casualty's heart stops, or has stopped beating, you must perform External Chest Compression in conjunction with Mouth-to-Mouth Ventilation. This is because without the heart to circulate the blood, oxygenated blood cannot reach the casualty's brain.

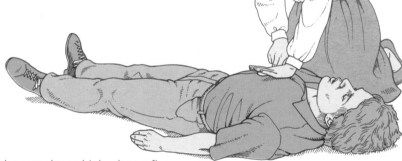

1 Lay the casualty on his back on a firm surface. Kneel alongside him facing his chest and in line with his heart. Find the junction of his rib margins at the bottom of his breastbone. Place the heel of one hand along the line of the breastbone, two finger breadths above this point, keeping your fingers off the ribs.

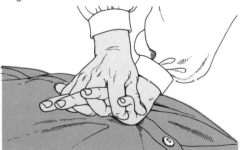

2 Cover this hand with the heel of your other hand and interlock your fingers. Your shoulders should be directly over the casualty's breastbone and your arms straight.

THE CORRECT POSITION FOR THE HAND

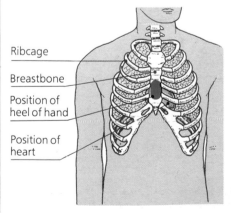

Ribcage

Breastbone

Position of heel of hand

Position of heart

It is most important that pressure from your hands is applied in the exact position shown.

3 Keeping your arms straight, press down vertically on the lower half of his breastbone to move it 4–5 cm (1½–2 in) for the average adult. Release pressure. Complete 15 compressions at the rate of 80 compressions per minute. Compressions should be regular and smooth, not jerky and jabbing. (To find the correct speed, count one and two and three, and so on.)

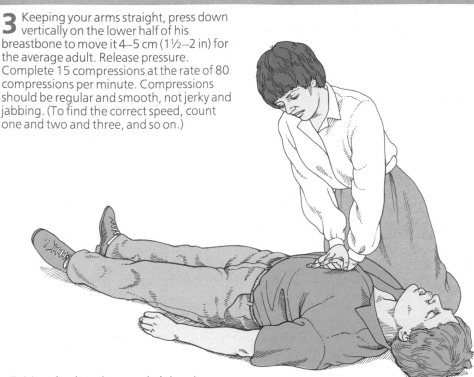

4 Move back to the casualty's head, re-open his airway, and give two breaths of Mouth-to-Mouth Ventilation.

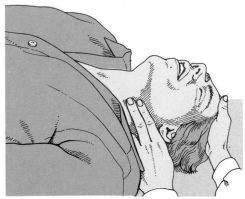

5 Continue with 15 compressions followed by two full ventilations, repeating the circulation check after the first minute. Thereafter, check pulse after every three minutes.

6 As soon as the pulse returns, stop compressions immediately. Continue Mouth-to-Mouth Ventilation until natural breathing is restored, assisting it when necessary, and adjusting it to the casualty's rate. Place the casualty in the Recovery Position (see p.24).

CHECKING FOR RESPONSE
When resuscitation is successful, the carotid pulse will return. Look at the casualty's face and lips. The colour will improve as blood containing oxygen begins to circulate. When the casualty is not breathing, the normal colour turns to blue (cyanosis).

RESUSCITATION WITH TWO FIRST AIDERS

When two First Aiders are present, one should take charge and maintain the open airway, perform Mouth-to-Mouth Ventilation and check circulation; the other should perform External Chest Compression. If resuscitation is prolonged, the First Aiders can change places to reduce the strain, and it may be easier if they work on opposite sides of the body.

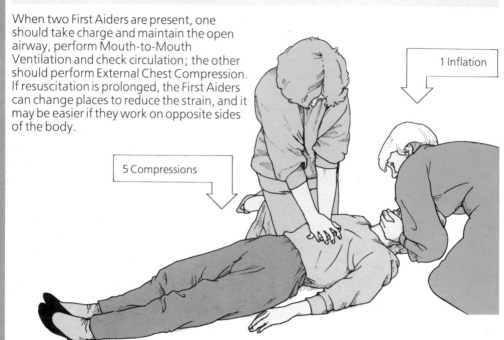

1 Inflation

5 Compressions

1 One First Aider takes up a position at the casualty's head, the other kneels alongside the casualty, level with the middle of her chest.

2 The First Aider at the head immediately opens the airway, gives the first two inflations and checks for circulation (see p.17). If it is absent, the other First Aider should begin chest compression.

3 Resuscitation then continues with the First Aider at the head keeping the airway open and giving a *single* inflation on the upstroke of every fifth compression by her partner. The compressions are continued at a rate of 80 per minute until the circulation returns and the pulse is felt. (To find the correct speed, count as on p.21.)
    Pulse check must be carried out after the first minute and then every three minutes.

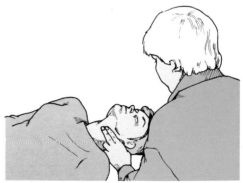

NOTE
There needs to be a short pause after every five compressions, allowing time for the lungs to inflate.

RESUSCITATION FOR CHILDREN

The techniques for resuscitating youths and older children are the same as for adults (see pp.18–21), but they must be done slightly faster and with lighter pressure. For children and infants place your hand just below the *centre* of the breastbone for External Chest Compression giving five compressions to one inflation per cycle.

ARTIFICIAL VENTILATION

For children Open the child's airway. Seal your lips around his mouth and nose and breathe gently into the lungs at a rate of 20 breaths per minute. Check for circulation after giving the first two inflations.

For babies or children under two Open the airway being careful *not* to tilt the head back too far. Seal your lips aroung the baby's *mouth and nose* and puff gently into the lungs at a rate of 20 breaths per minute. Check for circulation after giving the first two inflations.

IF it is difficult to feel the carotid pulse in an infant, check the brachial pulse. This is located on the inside of the upper arm, midway between shoulder and elbow. Place your thumb on the outside of the arm and your index and middle fingers on the inside. Press your fingertips lightly towards the bone.

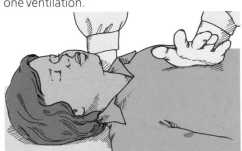

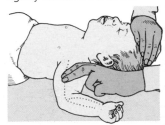

EXTERNAL CHEST COMPRESSION

For children Use light pressure with *one hand only*. Press at a rate of 100 compressions per minute to a depth of 2.5–3.5 cm (1–1½ in) with five compressions to one ventilation.

For babies or children under two Make sure the baby is on a firm surface. Support his head and neck by sliding one hand under his back. Using *two fingers only*, press at a rate of 100 times per minute to a depth of 1.5–2.5 cm (½–1 in).

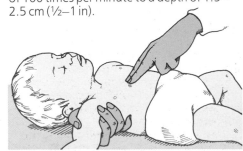

THE RECOVERY POSITION

Unconscious casualties who are breathing and whose hearts are beating should be placed in the *Recovery Position*. This position ensures that an open airway is maintained, because: the tongue cannot fall to the back of the throat; the head and neck will remain in an extended position so that the air passage is widened; and vomit or other fluid will drain freely from the casualty's mouth.

The position of the casualty's limbs provides the necessary stability to keep the body propped in a safe and comfortable position. Depending upon the injuries or condition, you may have to modify the technique in order to avoid causing further damage to injuries (see opposite).

The Recovery Position may not be an ideal position initially if you are examining a casualty or for the treatment of a spinal injury (see *Spinal Injury Recovery Position*, p.96). However, it *must* be used immediately if a casualty's breathing becomes difficult or noisy and is not relieved by opening the airway, or if a casualty has to be left unattended (an unusual event).

The technique shown here is the sequence for turning a casualty who is lying on his or her back; not all these steps will be necessary if he or she is lying on the side or front. If the casualty is wearing spectacles, these should be removed before turning the head to avoid eye injuries.

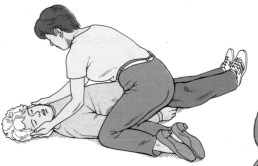

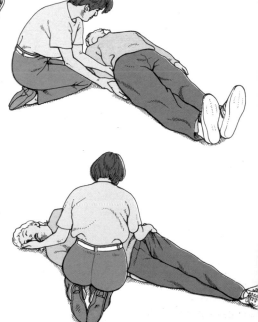

1 Kneel upright alongside the casualty facing his chest. Turn his head towards you and tilt it back keeping the jaw forward in the Open Airway Position (see p.14).

2 Place the casualty's arm nearest to you by his side. Lift his buttock and place his hand well underneath with the fingers straight. Holding his far leg under the knee or ankle bring it towards you and cross it over his near leg. Bring his other forearm over the front of his chest.

3 Protect and support the casualty's head with one hand. With the other hand, grasp his clothing at the hip furthest from you and pull him towards you. Support him on his side against your thighs.

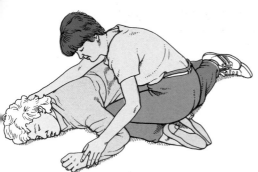

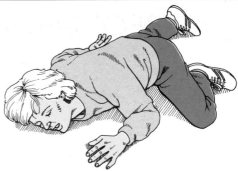

4 Still supporting his body against your knees, re-adjust his head to ensure that the airway is open.

5 Bend his uppermost arm at a right angle to support the upper body.

7 Carefully pull the other arm out from under the casualty, working from the shoulder down. Leave it lying parallel to him to prevent him rolling on to his back and to avoid interference with his circulation.

8 Check that the final position is stable and that the casualty cannot roll forwards or backwards. Ensure that no more than half his chest is in contact with the ground and that his head remains tilted and his jaw forward to maintain an open airway position.

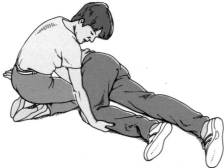

6 Bend his uppermost knee at a right angle to bring the thigh well forward to support the lower body.

FOR A HEAVY CASUALTY

You may have to use both hands to turn a heavy casualty. Grasp the clothing at the shoulders and hips and pull him so that his body is against your thighs.

If bystanders are present, one may support his head while you do the turning. Alternatively, get them to help by kneeling beside you and by pulling at his hips while you pull his shoulders and support his head. It may be necessary for them to face you and push the casualty towards you as you pull.

MODIFICATIONS

It may not be possible to follow the above procedure where there are fractures to the upper or lower body, when the casualty is lying in a confined space or if the bent limbs cannot be used as props. In such cases, the Recovery Position can be maintained by laying a rolled blanket down the front of the body. This method can also be used to transport a casualty on a stretcher in the Recovery Position. (For Spinal Injury Recovery Postion, see p.96.)

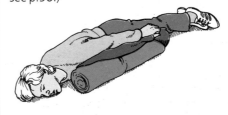

BLOOD & THE CIRCULATION

There are approximately six litres (10 pints) of blood in the normal adult's circulatory system. Blood carries oxygen and other nutrients to the tissues, and carbon dioxide and other waste products away from them. It flows through a network of flexible tubes called blood vessels. There are three different types — arteries, capillaries and veins.

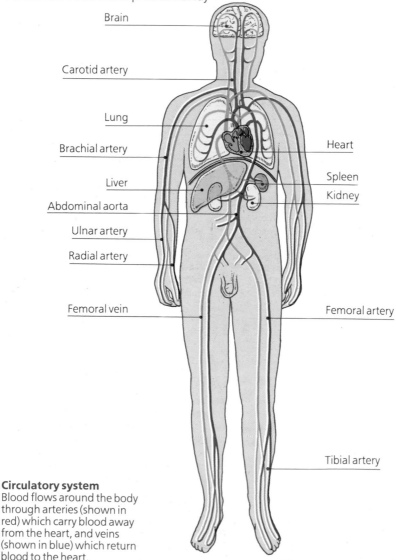

Brain

Carotid artery

Lung

Brachial artery

Heart

Liver

Spleen

Kidney

Abdominal aorta

Ulnar artery

Radial artery

Femoral vein

Femoral artery

Tibial artery

Circulatory system
Blood flows around the body through arteries (shown in red) which carry blood away from the heart, and veins (shown in blue) which return blood to the heart.

Arteries carry blood away from the heart. They are the strongest of the blood vessels and their walls contain elastic and muscular tissue. As the blood is forced along the arteries by the action of the heart, the muscular wall expands and then returns to its normal size. This wave of pressure is called the *pulse* and it can be felt wherever an artery is close to the surface and can be pressed against a bone, e.g., at the wrist (see p.85). Arteries divide becoming smaller and thinner as they reach the tissues until they become capillaries.

Capillaries are very small blood vessels, consisting only of a thin layer of cells through which the exchange of fluids and gases to and from the tissue cells of the body can be made. Having done this, the tiny capillaries gradually join up and become veins.

Veins carry blood back to the heart. Smaller veins unite, gradually becoming larger until they end in two large veins which return the blood to the right collecting chamber of the heart. Veins have little muscular tissue, and they rely on the squeezing action of the body muscles to make blood flow through them. Because of this, veins have one-way "cup-like" valves which help to control the flow of blood back to the heart.

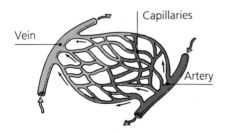

The network of blood vessels

Severe bleeding
When you cut yourself you bleed because pressure inside the blood vessels forces blood out. In arterial bleeding, bright red-coloured blood pumps out in time with the heart; in venous bleeding, the blood is a darker red and gushes out with less pressure; in capillary bleeding, blood oozes out.

The body contains certain inbuilt mechanisms to slow down or stop bleeding spontaneously. When a wound occurs the cut ends of a blood vessel contract to reduce the loss of blood and blood pressure falls. Blood clots form and plug up damaged vessels. The more slowly blood flows from a wound, the easier it is for a clot to form; the faster blood flows, the more likely it is that any clots will be washed away.

The dangers of blood loss
Normally the loss of a pint of blood in an adult is barely noticeable, but by the time that three pints, or about a third of the total blood volume is lost, the results can be serious because there is not enough left to provide a sufficient flow around the body. If you do not act quickly to stop severe bleeding there is a danger that shock (see p.86), and even loss of the casualty's life, may result.

The symptoms and signs of severe blood loss are due partly to the blood loss itself, and partly to the body's reaction to that loss; they may not all be apparent in every casualty. They are:
■ The face and lips become pale and the skin feels cold and clammy as the vessels which supply blood to the skin constrict in order to divert blood to the vital organs.
■ The pulse becomes faster to compensate for blood loss, but weaker.
■ The casualty may become anxious, restless and talkative.
■ He or she may feel thirsty due to the body's natural urge to replace lost fluid, and hunger for air to replace lost oxygen.
■ Blurring of vision, giddiness, clouding of consciousness and fainting due to a reduction in the flow of blood to the brain, particularly if bleeding is prolonged.

Act quickly to stop bleeding if:
■ A large amount of blood is being lost.
■ The bleeding appears to be arterial — bright red and spurting regularly.

CONTROLLING BLOOD LOSS

The principle of controlling blood loss is to restrict the blood flow to the wound and therefore encourage clotting. This is done in two ways – by *pressure* and by *elevation*. There are two kinds of pressure: direct pressure over the wound and indirect pressure on the artery which supplies the area. Direct pressure must always be applied first; only use indirect pressure if it fails or proves to be impossible.

DIRECT PRESSURE

In order to stop bleeding without interfering with the rest of the circulation, you should immediately apply pressure directly on the wound. This direct pressure flattens the blood vessels in the area and helps to slow down the flow of blood, so that clots can form. Pressure has to be maintained for 5–15 minutes because it takes time to halt the flow of blood. If there is a foreign body embedded in the wound, pressure has to be applied alongside it.

If possible, you should also raise the injured part and support it in this position. This will slow down the flow of blood by lowering the local blood pressure.

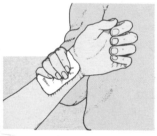

Apply direct pressure even if no dressing is available. If the wound is gaping, squeeze the edges together, gently but firmly.

IF the casualty is capable, ask him to apply direct pressure.

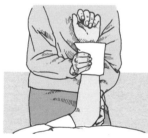

1 Cover the wound with a sterile dressing and apply direct pressure with your thumb and/or fingers.

2 Lay the casualty down in a suitable and comfortable position. Raise the injured part as far as possible and support it.

3 Apply a sterile dressing and sufficient padding to extend well beyond the edges of a wound and, in the case of a limb, to encircle it.

IF no sterile dressing is available, an improvised dressing can be made from any suitable clean material (see p.172).

IF bleeding continues, apply further padding and bandage firmly. Do not remove the original dressing as this may disturb clots and restart the bleeding.

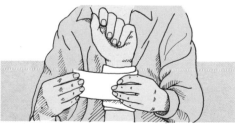

4 Press the padding down and secure with a bandage tied firmly enough to control bleeding, but not so tight as to cut off circulation (see p.175). Immobilize injured part (see *Fractures*, pp.106–123).

INDIRECT PRESSURE

If bleeding cannot be controlled by direct pressure or if it is impossible to apply direct pressure successfully (for example, if there are severe lacerations), you may be able to control it by applying indirect pressure at the appropriate pressure point. However, this method can only be used to control arterial bleeding from a limb.

A pressure point is the place where you can compress an artery against an underlying bone to flatten it and prevent the flow of blood beyond that point. However, since this cuts off the supply of blood to the tissues of the entire limb, *this method should only be used as a last resort and must not be applied for longer than 15 minutes.*

There are two pressure points used to control severe bleeding, one is on the *brachial* artery in the arm, and the other is on the *femoral* artery in the groin.

The brachial artery runs along the inner side of the upper arm between the muscles and its course roughly follows the seam of the sleeve. To apply pressure, place your hands under the casualty's arm and slide your fingers between the muscles. Press upwards and inwards pushing the artery against the bone.

The femoral artery passes into the lower limb at a point corresponding to the centre of the fold of the groin and runs along the inside of the thigh. To apply pressure, lay the casualty down with knee bent. Locate the artery in the groin and press it against the underlying bone with your thumbs, fist or heel of your hand.

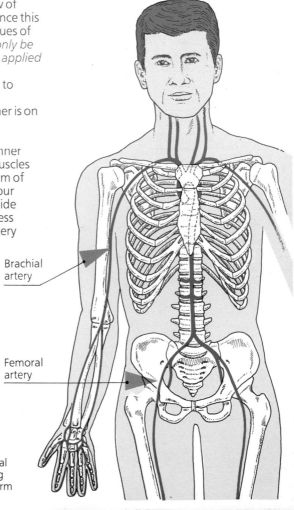

Brachial artery

Femoral artery

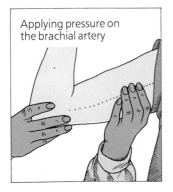

Applying pressure on the brachial artery

Pressure points
Compressing either the brachial or femoral arteries by pressing against the underlying bone will cut off the blood supply to the arm or leg respectively.

ACTION AT AN EMERGENCY

The basic principles of First Aid apply to all injuries or illnesses regardless of severity. Whatever the incident, it is the First Aider's responsibility to act quickly, calmly and correctly in order to:

- Preserve life.
- Prevent deterioration in the casualty's condition.
- Promote recovery.

These objectives are best achieved by:

- A rapid but calm approach.
- A quick assessment of the situation and the casualty.
- A correct diagnosis of the condition based on the history of the incident, and the casualty's history, symptoms and signs.
- Immediate and appropriate treatment of any conditions diagnosed.
- Proper disposal of the casualty according to the injury or condition.

APPROACH

This should be speedy but calm and controlled. Ensure that you are not placing yourself in any danger when approaching the casualty. On arrival at the scene of any incident, state that you are a trained First Aider and, if there are no doctors, nurses or more experienced people present, calmly take charge.

General rules
Whenever and wherever you come across an emergency, use your common sense, know your limitations and do not attempt to do too much.

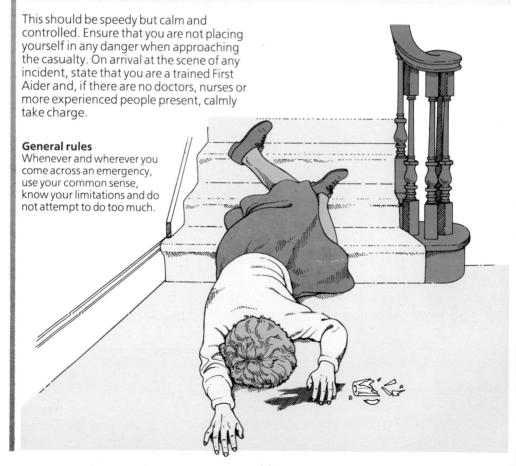

ASSESSING THE SITUATION

As soon as you have taken control at an incident, it is crucial that you make an accurate assessment of the situation and decide on the priorities of action. To do this you must consider: whether you and the casualty are in any danger; if the casualty has any life-threatening conditions; if any bystanders can help you; and whether you need to call for assistance.

SAFETY

You must minimize the risk of danger to yourself, the casualty and any bystanders, and guard against any further casualties arising. For example, in the case of:

■ **Road accidents** Instruct a bystander to control the traffic, keeping it well away from yourself and the casualty. Watch out for fire risks, especially from petrol spillage and switch off the ignition of the vehicles concerned (see p.165).

■ **Gas and poisonous fumes** If possible, cut off the source, and ensure adequate ventilation.

■ **Electrical contact** Break the contact, if possible, and take the necessary precautions against further contact.

■ **Fire and collapsing buildings** Move the casualty to safety immediately if you can do so without endangering your own life.

GETTING OTHERS TO HELP YOU

Some bystanders can be extremely useful and may be able to assist with treatment — for example, controlling severe bleeding or supporting a badly injured limb. Other bystanders may become nuisances so you must keep them occupied to prevent them interfering with your work. They can be asked to control traffic or crowds, or be sent to telephone for assistance (see p.32). However, when sending bystanders to the telephone make sure that they understand the message that is to be sent. If possible, ask them to write it down but, in any case, ask them to repeat the message to you before actually sending it. Always make sure that they report back to you afterwards.

DETERMINING PRIORITIES

In order to determine the condition of a casualty, ask him "what happened?". A reply will help you to know what to look for. It also tells you that: he is conscious; his airway is clear; he is able to breathe. If he does not respond to questioning or touch, perform the following checks immediately.

Airway, breathing and circulation
Following the ABC rule (see p.10), quickly check that the **airway** is open (see p.14) and that the casualty is **breathing**. If not, commence Artificial Ventilation immediately (see p.18). Check pulse for **circulation** (see p.17). If absent, commence External Chest Compression (see p.21). Check for any severe bleeding and control it (see p.28).

Unconsciousness
Place an unconscious casualty, or one whose breathing is noisy, in the Recovery Position (see p.24) and assess the level of responsiveness (see p.95). If there is any possibility of spinal injury, do not turn him (see p.96), unless difficulty in breathing makes it essential, or vomiting is likely to occur.

Shock
Keep the casualty warm, quiet and lying down until skilled help arrives (see p.86).

Other needs
Unless there is immediate danger to life from the surroundings treat all fractures and large wounds before moving a casualty. If the casualty is in danger, support the injured part whilst moving (see *Fractures*, pp.106–123). If you suspect that the casualty has a fractured spine, see pp.96 and 125.

CALLING FOR ASSISTANCE

Once you decide that assistance is required, and this may include ambulance, police, fire brigade, gas or electricity boards, send for it immediately. Go to the nearest telephone, or send a bystander, dial 999 and state the service required, normally ambulance. Do not leave the casualty unattended.

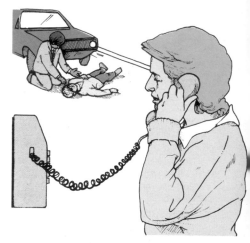

Whether you are giving the message yourself or instructing someone to do so make sure that the following information is passed on:

1 Your telephone number (if for any reason you are cut off the officer will then be able to contact you).

2 The exact location of the incident; if you can, point out nearby road junctions or other landmarks.

3 An indication of the type and seriousness of the incident, e.g., "Road traffic accident, two cars involved, three people trapped".

4 The number, sex and approximate age of the casualties involved and, if possible, the nature of their injuries.

5 Request special aid if you suspect a heart attack or childbirth.

DO NOT replace the receiver before the control officer does so.

NOTE
Each control officer has direct access to the other emergency switchboards and will pass on any messages, if necessary.

MULTIPLE CASUALTIES & INJURIES

Where there is more than one casualty, you must decide by rapid assessment which one needs priority of treatment. Remember that the noisiest casualty is rarely the most severely injured.

In First Aid, common sense is almost as important as the actual knowledge of the subject. In real life, serious accidents rarely produce only a single injury. Frequently two or more injuries occur so that the correct treatment of one may interfere with the correct treatment of the other. In such circumstances, you must decide which injury is the more serious and treat that one in the correct way. You should then deal with the other injuries as correctly as possible under the conflicting circumstances.

EXAMINATION & DIAGNOSIS

Having dealt with the priorities (see p.31), you should next attempt a fuller examination and diagnosis. This takes account of the casualty's *history* (and that of the incident), the *symptoms, signs* and *levels of responsiveness.*

History

This is the full story of how the incident occurred or the illness began, and should be taken directly from the casualty and a responsible bystander wherever possible. For example, a casualty may only say "I slipped and fell down" whereas a witness may say "I saw the old man fall and his head hit the wall". Pay full attention to the story, as it may provide clues to the likely injuries – especially if you suspect an existing illness such as diabetes or heart disease. Make a note of details of similar occurrences and treatments administered in the past for the examining doctor's benefit later.

Never hurry the casualty and remember to pass on all the information you have obtained when skilled help arrives.

Symptoms

These are sensations that the casualty feels and describes to you – the most useful of these is pain.

If the casualty is *conscious*, ask if there is any pain and, if so, where. Examine that part first, then run through the various sites at which pain is felt. Remember, however, that a severe pain in one area may mask a more serious injury, which produces less pain, in another. Other useful symptoms the casualty may disclose are nausea, giddiness, feelings of heat and cold, thirst, weakness or loss of muscular control or sensation. All symptoms should then be investigated and confirmed by a physical examination for signs of abnormality, such as injury or illness.

If the casualty is *unconscious*, or unreliable because dazed or in shock, then diagnosis cannot be based on symptoms but has to be based on information obtained from bystanders and *signs*.

Signs

These are details ascertained by you using your senses – sight, touch, hearing and smell. These may be: signs of injury such as bleeding, swelling, deformity or signs of illness such as a raised temperature and/or a rapid or an irregular pulse.

All these signs may be immediately obvious, noticed incidentally or deliberately discovered by a physical examination.

HOW TO CARRY OUT AN EXAMINATION

A general examination should be carried out quickly to discern any imminent threats to life whether the casualty is conscious or unconscious. When examining a casualty there are certain rules you should follow. These are:
■ Move him or her as little as possible to avoid aggravating any injuries.
■ Begin your examination at the head and work methodically towards his or her feet.
■ Remember to use all your senses – look, feel, listen and smell.

■ Always compare one side of the casualty's body with the other as this makes it easier to detect any swellings or irregularities that require first aid.

NOTE
If at any stage during the examination the casualty's breathing becomes noisy and difficult, place the casualty in the Recovery Position (see p.24).

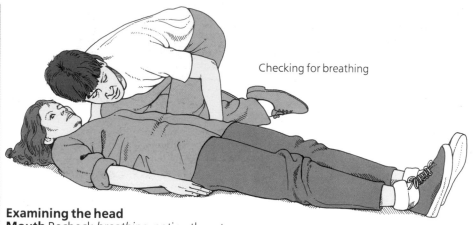

Checking for breathing

Examining the head

Mouth Recheck *breathing*, noting the rate, depth, and nature (whether easy or difficult, noisy or quiet); note also any *odour*. Check

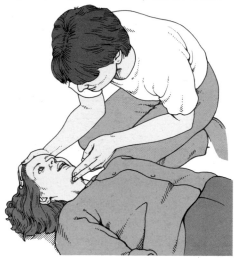

Looking for foreign bodies

the inside of the mouth to ensure it contains no foreign matter, such as vomit, blood, food, loose teeth, that might cause choking. Examine the *lips* for any signs of burning or discoloration that might indicate corrosive poisoning. Look inside the lips for blueness which might indicate asphyxia. Check the *teeth* to make sure that any recently dislodged teeth have not fallen down into the back of the throat. Make sure that dentures are firm-fitting (essential for resuscitation); if they are not remove them.

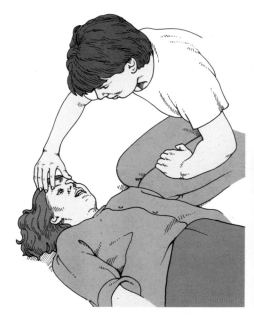

Examining the eyes

Eyes Examine both together comparing the pupils (the black circular centres) and noting whether they are equal in size. Check the white orb of the eye for bloodshot appearance.

Nose Check for signs of blood, clear fluid or a mixture of both which might come from inside the skull.

Face Look at the *colour* – it may be pale, flushed, or even bluish if breathing is affected. At the same time, feel the *temperature* of the face to check whether it is particularly hot or cold and note the state of the *skin* – whether it is dry or clammy or even sweating profusely.

Ears Check the ears for foreign bodies and traces of blood and/or clear cerebro-spinal fluid that might indicate skull fracture. Speak into the casualty's ears to test hearing.

Skull Gently run the hands over the scalp searching for bleeding, swelling or any indentation that might indicate a fracture.

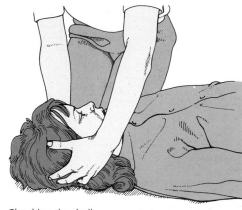

Checking the skull

Examining the neck and spine

Loosen clothing around the neck. Run your fingers over the spine from the base of the skull down to as far as you can reach between the shoulders, checking for any irregularity of the *vertebrae* that might indicate a fracture. Check round the neck, to see whether any warning *medallion* is being worn. Check the *carotid pulse*, and note its rate, strength and rhythm (see p.85). Note the presence or absence of movement or feeling in the casualty's limbs.

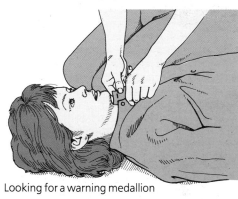

Looking for a warning medallion

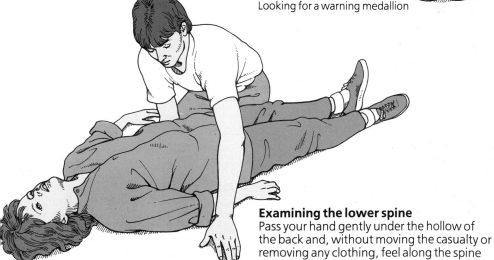

Examining the spine

Examining the lower spine

Pass your hand gently under the hollow of the back and, without moving the casualty or removing any clothing, feel along the spine as high and as low as you can checking for irregularity of the vertebrae or swelling.

Examining the trunk

Check the *chest* for evenness of rib movement on breathing and note any wounds that are "sucking" air (see p.76). Check the *ribs* for irregularity or depression that might indicate a fracture and also feel along the line of the *breastbone*.

Check both *collar-bones* for irregularity and the *shoulders* for signs of deformity. Carefully feel either side of the *pelvis* looking for signs of fracture and note any indication of *incontinence*.

Examining the arms

Examine the *upper-arm bones*, then the bones in the *forearm, wrists, hands* and *fingers*. Check carefully for any deformity and swelling which might indicate fractures. Check the forearms to see if the casualty is wearing a medical warning bracelet and for injection marks. Needle marks might indicate either drug abuse (see p.155) or diabetes (see p.105).

Examining the legs

Check the *hips, thighs, kneecaps*, both bones of the *lower legs*, the *ankles, feet* and *toes* in the same way as the arms.

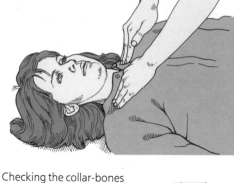

Checking the collar-bones

Examining the ribs

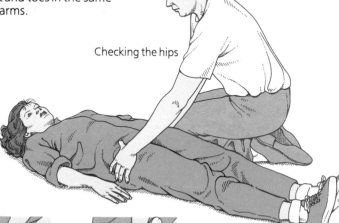

Checking the hips

Examining the knees   Checking the ankles

NOTE
Use two hands so that you can examine and compare both sides of the body at the same time.

LEVELS OF RESPONSIVENESS

There are various stages through which a casualty may pass during progression from consciousness to unconsciousness. These are dealt with in detail on p.95 but, basically, if the casualty responds well to stimuli then unconsciousness is only light (as in a faint, for example). However, he or she is still in a potentially dangerous state. If the response is poor or absent, the unconsciousness is deeper and the risk correspondingly greater.

Every 10 minutes you should recheck and note the casualty's response to the stimuli of *noise* (speak loudly into the ear), *touch* (try to arouse by shaking the shoulders gently) and *pain* (watch the face while you pinch the skin on hand or ankle). In addition, you should keep a similar check on the casualty's breathing (see p.15), pulse (see p.85) and temperature where appropriate (see pp.146 and 149). Your findings should be recorded.

AIDS TO DIAGNOSIS

Your diagnosis will be based on information from various sources. By taking the history of the incident, asking the casualty for symptoms and examining him or her for signs, it should be possible to make an accurate diagnosis. The following chart is a summary of how to achieve this.

HISTORY This is obtained from surroundings, casualty and bystanders.		
SYMPTOMS	**SIGNS**	
These are the sensations experienced by the casualty and obtained by asking tactful questions.	These are noted by the First Aider, using his or her own senses.	
Pain Loss of normal movement Loss of sensation Cold Heat Thirst Nausea Weakness Dizziness Faintness Temporary loss of consciousness Loss of memory Sensation of breaking bone	**SIGHT** Respiration Bleeding (type and volume) Wounds Foreign bodies Colour of face Swelling Deformity Bruising Reflexes Responses to touch and sound Incontinence Vomit Needle marks Containers **HEARING** Breathing Groans Crepitus (see p.108)	**TOUCH** Dampness (bleeding, incontinence) Temperature Pulse Swelling Deformity Irregularity Tenderness **SMELL** Breath Burning Gas Alcohol

EXTERNAL CLUES

If a casualty is unconscious, check their *pockets, handbag* or *briefcase* for possible clues. *Appointment cards* for a hospital or clinic or *information cards* may reveal that the casualty is on steroids or insulin or is liable to epileptic fits (see p.102). Lumps of sugar or glucose present may even indicate that the casualty is a diabetic (see p.105).

There are a number of *medical warning items* worn by those with a medical condition. They may take the form of an inscribed medallion or bracelet

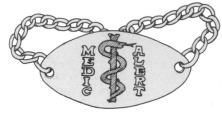

("Medic-alert", for example), a locket for wrist or neck or a capsule on a neck chain or key-ring containing a strip of paper describing the casualty's condition.

TREATMENT

Carry out the appropriate treatment for each condition found, gently and quickly. It is most important that you reassure and encourage the casualty constantly. Work calmly and efficiently, pay attention to any remarks or requests that the casualty makes, and do not pester with questions. This is annoying for the casualty and is a sign of uncertainty on your part. After giving the necessary treatment, place the casualty in the appropriate position and keep a watchful eye until help arrives.

Bear in mind your aim is to preserve life, prevent the condition worsening and promote recovery.

breathing and the heart is not beating, and continue treatment until skilled medical aid is available.
■ Control bleeding.

To prevent the condition worsening
■ Dress wounds.
■ Provide comfortable support for any large wounds and fractures.
■ Place the casualty in the most comfortable position consistent with the requirements of treatment.

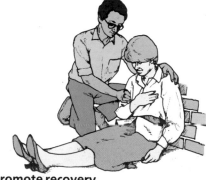

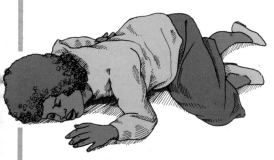

To preserve life
■ Maintain an open airway by positioning the casualty correctly.
■ Begin resuscitation if the casualty is not

To promote recovery
■ Relieve the casualty of anxiety and encourage confidence.
■ Attempt to relieve the casualty of pain and discomfort.
■ Handle the casualty gently.
■ Protect the casualty from the cold and wet.

AFTER TREATMENT

Once you have carried out your treatment the casualty should normally receive attention from a qualified person (doctor or nurse) without undue delay. Depending on the severity of the condition and the availability of skilled help you should:

1 Arrange transport to hospital by ambulance (or by car for minor injuries and arm fractures).

2 Hand over the casualty to the care of a doctor or nurse at the scene.

3 Take the casualty to a nearby house or shelter to await the arrival of the ambulance or doctor.

4 Allow the casualty to go home and advise him or her to seek medical advice, if necessary.

NOTE
Never send anyone home who has been unconscious, even for a short time, or who is in shock; seek medical aid.

MAKING A REPORT

The casualty should always be accompanied by a brief written report when he or she leaves your care. If necessary, you should accompany the casualty yourself and make a personal report.
   The need to supply complete information cannot be emphasized enough, and it should include the following:
■ History of the accident or illness.
■ Brief description of the injury.
■ The level of responsiveness and any changes.
■ Any other associated injuries.
■ The pulse and any changes.
■ The skin colour and any changes.
■ Blood loss sustained.
■ Any unusual behaviour by the casualty.
■ Any treatment given and when.

Informing relatives
You should also send a tactful message to the casualty's home stating what has happened and where he or she has been taken if this has not already been done by the police or other authority attending the incident. If the casualty is unconscious or unable to tell you where to contact his

relatives, look for a diary or donor card which may give the relevant details (see *External Clues*, opposite).

Property
Take care of any property belonging to the casualty and hand it over to the police or ambulance personnel.

REMOVING CLOTHING

Sometimes it is necessary to remove clothing in order to expose injuries, make an accurate diagnosis or conduct a proper treatment. This should be done with the minimum of disturbance to the casualty, and you should only remove as much as is actually necessary. Clothing should not be damaged unnecessarily. If very tight underclothing, such as a girdle, has to be cut, do this along the seams, if it is possible. Maintain sufficient privacy.

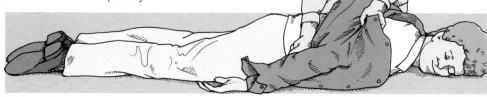

Removing a coat or jacket
Raise the casualty and slip the garment over his shoulders. Bend his arm on the sound side and remove the coat from that side first. Then, slip the injured arm out of its sleeve, keeping the arm straight if possible. If necessary, slit up the seam on the casualty's injured side.

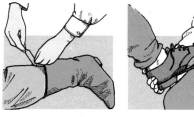

Removing a shirt or vest
Remove as for a coat. If necessary, slit it down the front or side.

Removing boots or shoes
Support the ankle, undo or cut any laces and carefully remove the shoe. If the casualty is wearing long boots, that will not unfasten, carefully slit them down the back seam with a sharp knife.

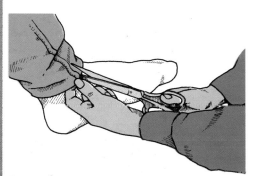

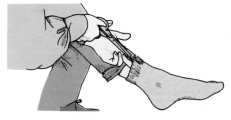

Removing trousers
Pull them down from the waist to reveal the casualty's thigh or raise the trouser leg to expose the calf and knee. If necessary, slit up the inside seam.

Removing socks
If these are difficult to remove, insert your first two fingers between the sock and the leg. Raise the sock and cut it between your fingers with scissors.

REMOVING CRASH-HELMETS

Whether or not you remove a protective helmet, such as a motorcycle crash-helmet, depends on the situation and condition of the casualty. *It is best left on and should only be removed if the casualty's condition warrants it.* If possible, the helmet should be removed by the casualty. A full-face helmet that encloses the head and face should *only* be removed if it obstructs breathing, if the casualty is vomiting or if there are severe head injuries.

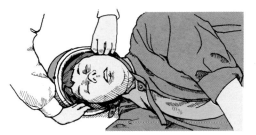

Removing an open-face helmet
Unfasten or cut through the chinstrap, if necessary. Take pressure off the head by forcing the sides apart, then lift the helmet upwards and backwards.

Removing a full-face helmet
To remove it safely, two people are needed, one to support the casualty's head and neck, while the other lifts the helmet.

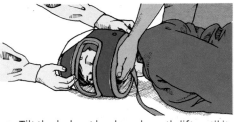

1 Tilt the helmet back and gently lift until it is clear of the chin.

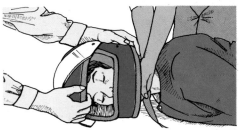

2 Tilt the helmet forward to pass over the base of the skull, then lift it straight off.

SUMMARY

■ Ensure that there is no further danger to the casualty or yourself.
■ Act quickly, quietly and methodically, giving priority to the urgent conditions.
■ If the casualty is unconscious, open the airway, check for breathing, and complete the ABC of Resuscitation if required, and place the casualty in the Recovery Position.
■ Control bleeding.
■ Minimize shock.
■ Determine the casualty's level of responsiveness.
■ Reassure the casualty to lessen anxiety.
■ Position the casualty correctly and comfortably but do not move more than is absolutely necessary.

■ Consider the possibility of internal bleeding and poisoning.
■ Treat large wounds and fractures before moving the casualty.
■ If necessary, arrange for urgent removal to hospital or into a doctor's care.
■ Watch and record any changes.
■ Do not attempt too much.
■ Do not allow people to crowd round; this hinders First Aid and may cause the casualty anxiety or embarrassment.
■ Do not remove clothing unnecessarily.
■ Do not attempt to give anything by mouth to a casualty who is unconscious, who has a suspected internal injury or who may shortly need an anaesthetic.

ASPHYXIA

This is a potentially fatal condition which occurs if there is not enough oxygen available to the tissues of the body. Such lack may be due to an insufficient amount of oxygen in the air breathed in or any interference with, or injury to, the respiratory system. Without an adequate supply of oxygen, the tissues deteriorate very rapidly: vital nerve cells in the brain can die after only three minutes without oxygen.

There are many conditions which can result in asphyxia, some of which are described below.

Conditions affecting the casualty's airway and lungs include:
■ *Obstructed airway* due to the tongue falling into the back of the throat in an unconscious casualty; food, vomit or other foreign matter present in the airway; or swelling of the tissues in the throat resulting from scalds, stings or infection.
■ *Fluid in the air passages.*
■ *Compression of the windpipe* by hanging or strangulation.
■ *Compression of the chest* caused by a fall of earth or sand, being crushed against a wall or barrier or pressure from a crowd.
■ *Injury to the lungs.*
■ *Injury to the chest wall*, e.g., a "stove-in-chest".
■ *Fits* preventing adequate breathing.

Conditions affecting the brain or nerves which control respiration include:
■ *Electrical injury.*
■ *Poisoning.*
■ *Paralysis* caused by a stroke or injury to the spinal cord.

Conditions affecting the amount of oxygen in the blood include:
■ *Air containing insufficient oxygen* such as may be found in gas or smoke-filled buildings or shafts and tunnels.
■ *Change in atmospheric pressure* at high altitudes, in depressurized aircraft or after deep sea diving.

Conditions preventing the use of oxygen in the body include:
■ *Carbon monoxide poisoning.*
■ *Cyanide poisoning.*

GENERAL SYMPTOMS & SIGNS
■ Difficulty in breathing: the rate and depth of breathing increases.
■ Breathing may become noisy with snoring or gurgling.
■ Possible frothing at the mouth.
■ Blueness of face, lips and fingernails (cyanosis).
■ Confusion.
■ Lowering of level of responsiveness.
■ Possible unconsciousness.
■ Breathing may stop.

AIM
Maintain or restore the casualty's breathing and seek medical aid.

GENERAL TREATMENT

1 Remove the cause of asphyxia and open the airway (see p.14). Ensure adequate fresh air.

2 If the casualty is unconscious, open her airway and check breathing. Complete the ABC of Resuscitation if required and place the casualty in the Recovery Position (pp.14–25).

3 Check breathing rate (see p.12), pulse rate (see p.85) and level of responsiveness (see p.95) at 10-minute intervals.

4 Seek medical aid as soon as possible.

SUFFOCATION (EXTERNAL OBSTRUCTION)

This results when air is prevented from reaching the air passages by an external obstruction such as a plastic bag, soft pillow or a fall of sand. (For suffocation by smoke, see p.46; for industrial gases, see p.157).

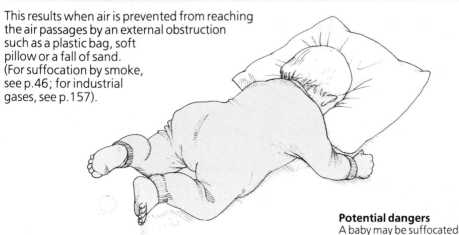

Potential dangers
A baby may be suffocated through lying face-down on a pillow or cushion.

SYMPTOMS & SIGNS
■ General symptoms and signs of asphyxia.

AIM
Restore supply of air to the casualty and seek medical aid.

TREATMENT

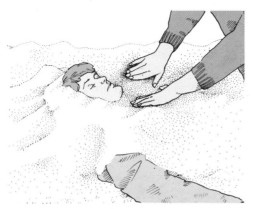

1 Immediately remove any obstruction or remove the casualty to fresh air.

2 If she is conscious and breathing, reassure and observe.

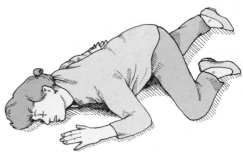

3 If she is unconscious, open her airway and check breathing. Complete the ABC of Resuscitation if required and place her in the Recovery Position (see pp.14–25).

4 Seek medical aid. If in doubt about her condition, arrange removal to hospital.

HANGING, STRANGLING & THROTTLING

Pressure on the outside of the neck by hanging, strangling or throttling squeezes the airway shut and blocks off the flow of air to the lungs. *Hanging* involves suspension of the body by the neck from a noose. *Strangling* involves cutting off the air supply by a tight constriction around the neck. *Throttling* involves cutting off the air supply by intentional squeezing of the person's throat, as in an assault. The first two conditions may occur accidentally, e.g., a tie may become caught in machinery.

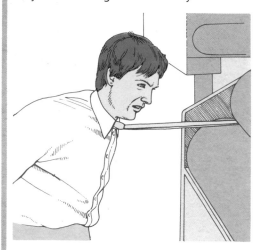

SYMPTOMS & SIGNS

- Body may still be suspended.
- General symptoms and signs of asphyxia.
- Congestion of the face and neck with the veins becoming prominent.
- Constriction may still be visible around neck (e.g., a scarf), or it may be hidden in the folds of the skin (e.g., wire).
- There may be marks around the casualty's throat or neck where a constriction has been removed.

AIM

Restore adequate breathing and arrange removal to hospital.

TREATMENT

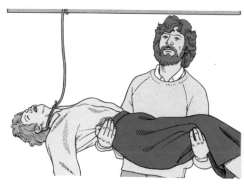

1 Remove the constriction from around the casualty's neck immediately, supporting the weight of her body if she is hanging.

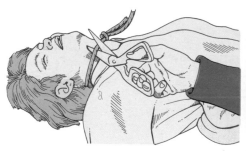

IF there is a knot, cut *below* it (a knot is difficult to cut and it may be useful evidence).

2 If the casualty is unconscious, open her airway and check breathing. Complete the ABC of Resuscitation if required and place the casualty in the Recovery Position (see pp.14–25).

3 Arrange removal to hospital.

NOTE
Seek medical aid even if recovery seems complete.

DROWNING

Drowning causes asphyxia by water entering the lungs or by causing the throat to go into spasm, so constricting the air passage (dry drowning). Do not waste time trying to remove any water from the casualty's lungs.

Congestion of the lungs can occur very quickly, but it may be several hours before it is apparent. *All casualties rescued from drowning should be sent to hospital.*

If a casualty has been immersed in cold water there is also a danger of hypothermia (see p.146), so it is important that the casualty is kept warm. (However, severe chilling protects the brain so that a casualty who has suffered prolonged immersion in very cold water may make a full recovery.)

SYMPTOMS & SIGNS

■ General symptoms and signs of asphyxia.
■ Froth around the casualty's lips, mouth and nostrils.

AIM

Get air into the casualty's lungs as fast as possible, in the water, if necessary. Arrange removal to hospital.

TREATMENT

1 Quickly remove any obstructions such as seaweed from the casualty's mouth and begin Artificial Ventilation immediately (see p.18). If he is still in the water, it may be possible to begin ventilation there.

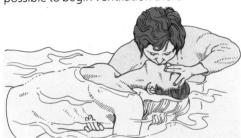

IF *within your depth* use one arm to support the casualty's body and use your other hand to support his head and seal his nose while you perform Mouth-to-Mouth Ventilation.

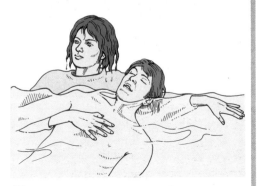

IF *in deeper water* give the occasional breath of air while towing the casualty ashore.

2 When you can place him on a firm surface, check breathing (see p.15) and pulse (see p.17), and continue resuscitation if necessary (pp.18–21).

3 As soon as the casualty begins breathing, place in the Recovery Position (see p.24).

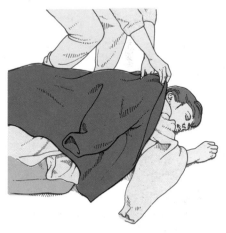

4 Keep him warm. If possible, remove wet clothing and dry him off. Cover with spare clothes and/or towels and, if necessary, treat for hypothermia (see p.146).

5 Arrange removal to hospital. Transport as a stretcher case, maintaining the treatment position.

SMOKE INHALATION

A fire uses up oxygen in the atmosphere so the oxygen level in a burning room is low and asphyxia may result. Smoke may irritate the throat, which can go into spasm and close the airway. In addition, the plastic coverings and foam padding of modern furnishings, when burning, often give off highly toxic fumes, which can be fatal.

SYMPTOMS & SIGNS
- General symptoms and signs of asphyxia.
- Casualty may be scorched or burned (scorched hair in the nostrils is a valuable warning sign).
- Symptoms and signs of shock brought on by burns (see p.86).

AIM
Restore fresh air and adequate breathing. Call the emergency services immediately. Remove the casualty from the fire and smoke if you can be sure there are *no* toxic fumes present. Try to extinguish the fire, and arrange removal to hospital.

TREATMENT

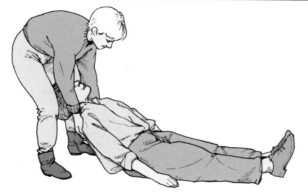

1 Remove the casualty to safety without endangering yourself (see p.168).

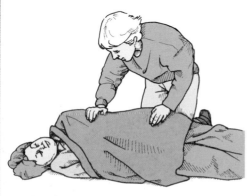

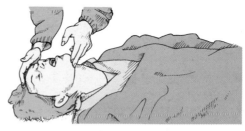

3 If she is unconscious, open her airway and check breathing. Complete the ABC of Resuscitation if required and place her in the Recovery Position (see pp.14–25).

4 Treat any burns (see *Burns & Scalds*, pp.137–139).

5 Arrange removal to hospital.

2 Extinguish any clothing that is on fire or smouldering (see p.137).

46

CARBON MONOXIDE POISONING

Carbon monoxide is a colourless, odourless gas. Its fumes are dangerous because carbon monoxide replaces the oxygen in the blood (it is more readily absorbed by the blood than is oxygen). A casualty may require prolonged Artificial Ventilation to clear it completely.

The most common sources of carbon monoxide are fumes from partially burnt fuels and motor engine exhausts. Danger arises if an exhaust system is defective or if an engine is left running in an enclosed space.

Enter a gas-filled room to rescue a casualty only if you are not in any danger and if you can get out again easily. Make sure you have back-up help. A rescue rope around the waist is a useful precaution.

SYMPTOMS & SIGNS

■ General symptoms and signs of asphyxia.
■ Casualty may complain of a headache.
■ Colour may be normal but will deepen to cherry pink as the level of carbon monoxide in the blood rises.
■ Casualty may be confused and unco-operative.
■ Breathing is difficult or may have stopped.
■ Unconsciousness may develop.

AIM

Restore fresh air and adequate breathing. Arrange removal to hospital.

TREATMENT

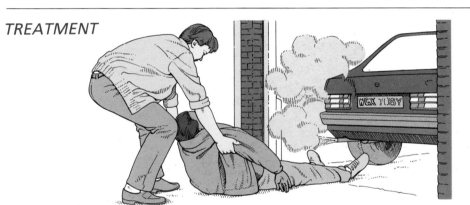

1 Open any doors and drag the casualty to safety if possible.

2 If the casualty is unconscious, open his airway and check breathing. Complete the ABC of Resuscitation if required and place the casualty in the Recovery Position (see pp.14–25).

3 Check breathing rate (see p.12), pulse (see p.85) and level of responsiveness (see p.95) at 10-minute intervals.

4 Arrange removal to hospital.

NOTE

There are many other gases which are dangerous because, although they are not toxic, they displace oxygen. *Carbon monoxide* is produced by the incomplete combustion of any fuel and *carbon dioxide* may be found in mines and similar enclosed spaces. *Butane* and *propane* are used at home and in industry for heating, lighting or refrigerating, and can leak from faulty connections.

CHOKING

This occurs when the airway is partially or totally obstructed by something which, in the act of swallowing, goes into the windpipe rather than down the food passage (see p.11). However, choking can also be caused by muscular spasm. Adults may choke on pieces of food which have been inadequately chewed and hurriedly swallowed; children are at risk because they like putting objects inside their mouths.

It is imperative that any obstruction be removed as soon as possible. Encourage a conscious choking casualty to cough the obstruction out. If this does not work, attempt to dislodge it by bending the casualty over and back slapping. *Only* if this fails, try to force the remaining air out of the lungs by abdominal thrust (see p.51).

Choking caused by food entering the windpipe

Food blocking windpipe

Normal passage of food

Both these techniques can be used by any First Aider on any casualty (infant, child or adult) in any position (sitting, standing or lying down). Administer both back slaps and abdominal thrusts up to four times in a sequence but if the technique is successful, the full series does not have to be completed.

Always treat a casualty in the position found (unless he or she is unconscious, see opposite). If standing or sitting, treat as opposite; if the casualty is lying down or if you are smaller than the casualty, treat as described for an unconscious casualty. (For choking children and infants, see p.50.)

If the casualty becomes unconscious, you will have to perform Artificial Ventilation in order to try to blow air past the obstruction and into the lungs (see p.18); in an unconscious casualty the throat may relax sufficiently to allow air past the obstruction.

SYMPTOMS & SIGNS
■ General symptoms and signs of asphyxia.
■ Casualty will be unable to speak or breathe and may be gripping the throat. The most remarkable feature is that he or she will be completely silent.
■ Congestion of the face and neck with the veins becoming prominent; blueness of the lips and mouth.
■ Possible unconsciousness.

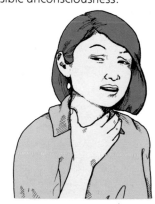

Casualty may grip throat

AIM
Remove the obstruction and restore normal breathing. Arrange removal to hospital.

TREATMENT

1 Remove any debris or false teeth from the casualty's mouth by hooking out with your fingers (see p.15), and encourage her to cough.

2 If the object is not dislodged by coughing, help the casualty to bend over with her head lower than her lungs. Slap her smartly between the shoulder-blades with the heel of your hand. Repeat up to four times if necessary.

3 Check her mouth to see if the obstruction has been dislodged. If it has not, you may be able to remove it by performing abdominal thrust (see p.51).

4 Check her mouth again. If the obstruction is visible but not coughed out, hook it out with your fingers.

5 If choking is not relieved, again repeat back slaps (up to four times) and abdominal thrusts (up to four times). If the casualty becomes unconscious, treat her as described below.

NOTE
The casualty may begin breathing again at any stage. When this happens advise the casualty to sit quietly and give sips of water as necessary.

FOR THE UNCONSCIOUS CHOKING CASUALTY

1 Turn the casualty on to her back, open her airway (see p.14) and begin Artificial Ventilation (see p.18).

2 If this is not successful, roll her on to the side facing you with her chest against your thigh and her head well back (see p.24), and perform up to four back slaps as described above.

3 Check the mouth to see if the obstruction has been dislodged. If it has, hook it out with your finger. If it has not, turn the casualty on to her back with her head in the Open Airway Position and perform abdominal thrust (see p.51).

4 Check the mouth again to see if the obstruction has been dislodged.

5 If choking persists, reposition the casualty's head and attempt Artificial Ventilation (see p.18). Then repeat steps 1–4 as necessary.

6 When the obstruction has been removed and the casualty is breathing, place her in the Recovery Position (see p.24) and arrange removal to hospital.

CHOKING FOR CHILDREN

Many children are comparable in height and build with small adults and can be treated in the same way using slightly less pressure. However, some modifications have to be made if you are treating a small child.

Follow the sequence described for adults but sit in a chair or kneel on one knee and lay the child over your knee, head down. Support the chest with one hand and slap the child smartly between the shoulder-blades up to four times with your other hand. If this does not dislodge the obstruction it may be necessary to perform abdominal thrust (see p.52).

If the child is or becomes unconscious, place on a firm surface and follow the sequence described for unconscious adults.

FOR INFANTS

The order of treatment for infants is the same as for children (see left) but *much* lighter presssure is used and the positions for back slapping and abdominal thrust are different.

Lay the infant's head downwards with the chest and abdomen lying along your forearm and use your arm to support the head and chest. Slap smartly between the shoulders up to four times. If this does not dislodge the obstruction, it may be necessary to perform abdominal thrust (see p.52).

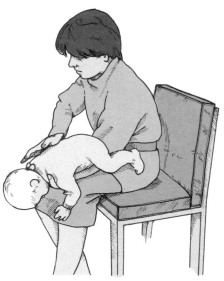

Treating a conscious choking infant

NOTE
Use extreme caution when removing an obstruction from the mouth of an infant. Only put your finger in the infant's mouth if you can see the obstruction and there is no danger of pushing the obstruction further down the infant's throat.

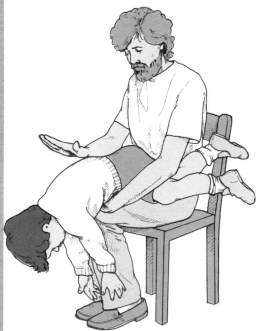

Treating a conscious choking child

ABDOMINAL THRUST

This is a technique which involves applying a series of thrusts to the upper abdomen in an attempt to force air out of a choking casualty's lungs. *Because there is a possibility that the action required can damage the underlying organs, abdominal thrust must only be used as a last resort after back slapping has failed.*

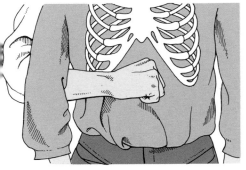

1 Stand or kneel behind the casualty and put one arm around her abdomen. Clench your fist and place it with your thumb inwards in the centre of her upper abdomen, between the navel and the breastbone.

2 Grasp your fist with your other hand.

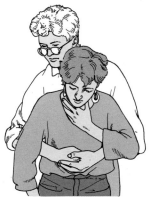

3 Pull both hands towards you with a quick inward and upward thrust from the elbows so that you compress the upper abdomen. The thrust must be hard enough to dislodge the obstruction. If it fails, repeat up to four times as necessary.

FOR THE UNCONSCIOUS CASUALTY

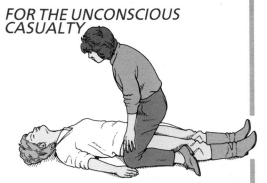

1 Turn the casualty on to her back with her head in the Open Airway Position (see p.14). Kneel astride her thighs so that you can apply sufficient pressure at the correct mid-abdominal position. If you cannot straddle her, kneel alongside.

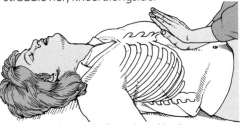

2 Place the heel of one hand in the centre of the casualty's upper abdomen and cover with your other hand, keeping fingers clear of her abdomen.

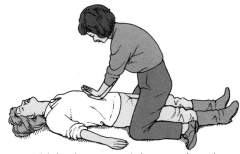

3 With both arms straight, press into the abdomen with a quick inward and upward thrust. The thrust must be hard enough to dislodge the obstruction. If it fails, repeat up to four times as necessary.

ABDOMINAL THRUST FOR CHILDREN

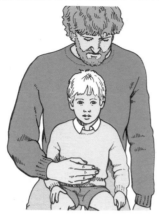

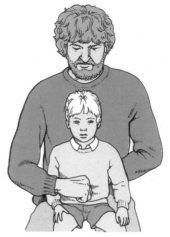

1 Sit the child on your lap or stand the child in front of you and place one arm around the abdomen.

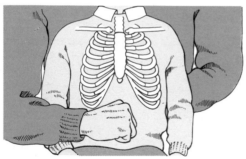

2 Clench your fist and place it with your thumb inwards in the centre of the upper abdomen, as on p.51. Support the back with your other hand.

3 Press your clenched fist into the abdomen with a quick inward and upward movement using much less pressure than for an adult. The thrust must be hard enough to dislodge the obstruction by itself. If it fails, repeat up to four times as necessary.

IF the child is unconscious, place in the same position as for an unconscious adult. Use the same method but only use one hand and apply less pressure.

FOR INFANTS
Place the infant on a firm surface with the head in the Open Airway Position (see p.14). Place the first two fingers of one hand on the upper abdomen, between the navel and the breastbone, and press with a quick inward and upward movement. The thrust must be hard enough to dislodge the obstruction. If it fails, repeat up to four times as necessary.

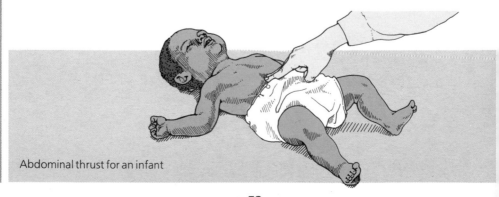

Abdominal thrust for an infant

BLAST INJURIES

Explosions can result from a bomb or if a flame or electrostatic discharge, from a doorbell or telephone for example, is introduced into an area where a combustible gas has been accumulating. The waves of high pressure from the blast may damage the lungs and other organs of the body.

The casualty may also be suffering from extensive burns, fractures, damaged eardrums, shock and other injuries due to flying glass or other debris.

SYMPTOMS & SIGNS
■ General symptoms and signs of asphyxia.
■ Casualty may cough up frothy, blood-stained spit.
■ Probability of multiple injuries.
■ Bleeding from the ear if the eardrum is damaged (see p.70).
■ Symptoms and signs of shock (see p.86).

AIM
Reassure the casualty and treat where found unless the possibility of further explosions exists. Arrange urgent removal to hospital.

TREATMENT

1 Reassure the casualty and move him as little as possible until a full examination reveals the extent of his injuries (see *Examination & Diagnosis*, pp.33–36).

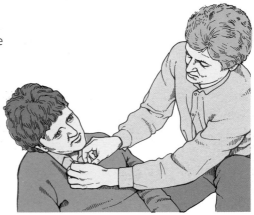

3 Loosen any constricting clothing around his neck, chest and waist.

4 Control bleeding and treat any wounds (see pp.62–65) or burns (see pp.137–139). Immobilize fractures (see pp.106–123).

5 Check breathing rate (see p.12), pulse (see p.85) and level of responsiveness (see p.95) at 10-minute intervals.

6 If the casualty is unconscious, open his airway and check breathing. Complete the ABC of Resuscitation if required and place the casualty in the Recovery Position (see pp.14–25).

7 Arrange urgent removal to hospital. Transport as a stretcher case, maintaining the treatment position.

2 If the casualty's general condition and injuries allow, raise him into a half-sitting position. Support his head and shoulders.

STOVE-IN-CHEST

Multiple fractures of the chest wall result in the area losing its rigidity and prevent it following the normal movements of the rib-cage during breathing (see p.12). Instead, the fractured ribs are sucked in during breathing-in and pushed out during breathing-out. This is a reversal of the normal movement of the ribcage and the opposite of what is happening on the sound side. This condition is known as *paradoxical breathing* and it may also inhibit the lung action on the uninjured side. In addition to this, the broken bones may damage other internal organs or penetrate the skin causing a "sucking" wound (see p.76).

Common causes of this type of injury are road traffic accidents in which the driver of a vehicle is thrown against the steering column or the steering column is pushed back into the driver's chest. The same effect can result if the chest is crushed by heavy objects.

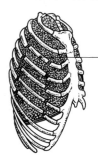

Multiple fractures

Severe chest injury
A blow to the chest may result in multiple fractures of the ribcage.

SYMPTOMS & SIGNS
■ General symptoms and signs of asphyxia.
■ Casualty finds it difficult and painful to breathe.
■ Casualty may be very distressed.
■ Unusual movement in the ribcage. Injured part of the chest wall may be seen to have lost rigidity.
■ Possibility of frothy blood-stained spit indicating lung damage (see *Penetrating Chest Wounds*, p.76).

AIM
Stabilize the chest wall to ease breathing. Arrange urgent removal to hospital.

TREATMENT
1 Support the affected part of the casualty's ribcage with your hand.

2 Help the casualty into a half-sitting position inclined towards the injured side. Support her head and shoulders.

3 Loosen any constricting clothing around her neck and waist.

4 If there is a "sucking" wound, treat it as on p.76.

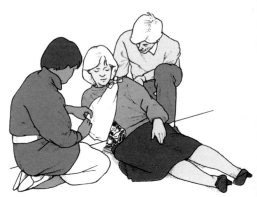

5 Immobilize the chest wall. Place a firm pad, e.g., a folded newspaper, over the injured area and place the arm on the injured side across the pad and support in an elevation sling (see p.179). If this is not sufficient to prevent the abnormal movement of the chest wall, apply a broad-fold bandage over the sling and right around the body; tie off in front on the uninjured side. If no bandage is available, use a scarf or belt.

6 Check for any signs of other injury.

7 If the casualty becomes unconscious, open her airway and check breathing. Complete the ABC of Resuscitation if required and place her in the Recovery Position with her sound side uppermost (see pp.14–25).

8 Arrange urgent removal to hospital. Transport as a stretcher case, maintaining the treatment position.

ASTHMA

Asthma is a distressing condition in which the muscles of the air passages go into spasm. The airway becomes constricted making breathing, particularly breathing out, very difficult. Asthma attacks can be triggered off by nervous tension or an allergy, although in many cases there is no obvious cause. Sudden attacks of difficult breathing sometimes occur at night. Regular asthma sufferers usually carry their own medication in the form of an aerosol to ease breathing in which case they will generally know how to cope with an attack.

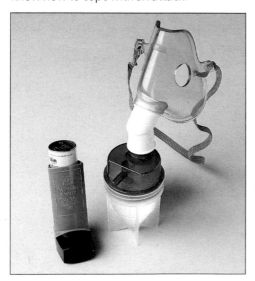

Medication for asthma sufferers
Regular sufferers may have an aerosol inhaler (left) or a nebulizer (right).

SYMPTOMS & SIGNS
■ Casualty may be very anxious and find it difficult to speak.
■ Difficulty in breathing, especially breathing out.
■ Blueness of the face.

AIM
Improve lung ventilation. Seek medical aid for prolonged or repeated attacks.

TREATMENT
1 Reassure and calm the casualty.

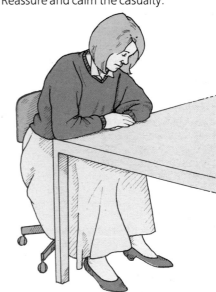

2 Advise her to sit down leaning slightly forward and rest on a support, e.g., a table. Ensure a good supply of fresh air.

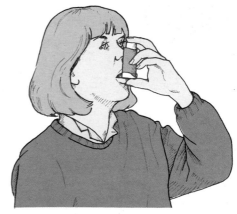

3 If the casualty has medication, allow her to take it because it may provide relief.

4 If the symptoms persist or recur, seek medical aid.

ELECTRICAL INJURIES

The passage of electrical current through the body may result in severe and sometimes fatal injuries. The current can come from a low or high voltage supply or lightning. The electricity can cause quivering of the heart muscle (fibrillation) or it can cause the heart to stop completely, which will also result in a cessation of breathing. The casualty may also have severe burns visible where the electricity enters the body as well as where it leaves the body to "earth", and there may be extensive internal damage between these points. The higher the voltage which passes through the body, the more extensive the burns will be.

Low-voltage appliances and cables in workshops, homes, offices and shops can cause electrical injuries. Most appliances and cables are insulated by non-conducting materials such as plastic or rubber to provide protection from the current. Many injuries result from faulty switches, frayed cables or defects within the appliances themselves. Young children are at risk because they may try to play with switches, wires and plugs.

Water is an excellent conductor of electricity, so that handling an otherwise safe appliance with wet hands or when standing on a wet floor substantially increases the risk of electrical injury.

Lightning is a natural source of electricity which can occur during a thunderstorm. It seeks contact with the ground through the nearest tall feature in the landscape. A person may be hit if in contact with, or standing near, isolated features such as trees, towers or pylons or simply by being the tallest feature in a flat area.

The current produced by lightning is of extremely short duration but it may set clothing on fire and stun the casualty. It can also cause instant death. You should always remove a casualty from a dangerous area as soon as possible.

Whatever the cause of the electrical injury, *never* touch the casualty with bare hands until you are sure that there is no further danger to yourself and that the casualty is no longer in contact with the source. In the case of injury from high-voltage electricity, do not approach the casualty until you are informed by the police or similar authority that it is safe to do so (see opposite).

SYMPTOMS & SIGNS

■ General symptoms and signs of asphyxia but the casualty's face may be ashen because breathing and heartbeat have stopped simultaneously.

■ Deep contact burns may be present at points of entry and exit.

■ Symptoms and signs of shock (see p.86).

AIM

Break the current or remove the casualty from the source if it is safe to do so. Arrange removal to hospital, if necessary.

TREATMENT

1 If the casualty is unconscious, open the airway and check breathing. Complete the ABC of Resuscitation if required and place the casualty in the Recovery Position (see pp.14–25).

2 Treat any burns (see pp.137–9, 143). Examine them carefully; they may be deeper than they appear at first.

3 To minimize shock, treat as on p.86.

4 Arrange removal to hospital in all cases where the casualty has required resuscitation, was unconscious, sustained burns or developed any of the symptoms and signs of shock.

NOTE
Pass on any information you have about the duration of electrical contact.

BREAKING A LOW-VOLTAGE CURRENT

Break the contact by switching off the current at the mains or meter if it can be quickly reached; if not, remove the plug or wrench the cable free.

If you cannot break the current, stand on some dry insulating material, such as a wooden box, rubber or plastic mat, or several layers of thick newspaper and, by means of a brush, wooden chair or stool, push the casualty's limbs away from the source.

Alternatively, loop a rope or tights around the casualty's feet or under the arms and pull him or her away from the source.

NOTE
Avoid using anything metallic or damp or allowing your hands to touch the casualty's flesh. If nothing else is available, pull his or her loose, dry clothing.

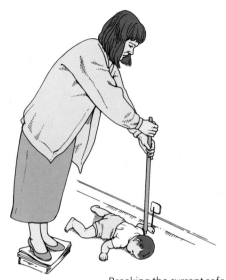

Breaking the current safely

INJURIES FROM HIGH-VOLTAGE ELECTRICITY

Contact with high-voltage currents found in power lines and overhead cables is usually immediately fatal. Severe burns always result and the force of sudden muscular spasm caused by the electricity may throw the casualty some distance from the point of contact and may cause fractures.

For safety, if a casualty remains in contact with, or is still within 18 m (20 yd) of, a high-current voltage, *never attempt to rescue or even approach* until the power has been cut off by the authorities. This is because the electricity may "arc" and jump considerable distances. Insulating material such as dry wood or clothing will not provide any protection.

Call the police immediately. Keep any bystanders away from the casualty and only give First Aid when you are officially informed that there is no further danger.

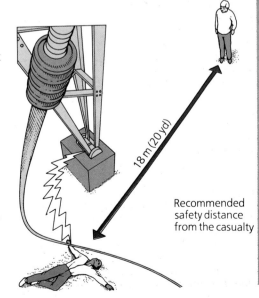

18 m (20 yd)

Recommended safety distance from the casualty

WINDING

A severe blow to or a heavy fall on the upper part of the abdomen (solar plexus) can upset the regularity of breathing.

SYMPTOMS & SIGNS
- General symptoms and signs of asphyxia, if prolonged.
- Difficulty in breathing in.
- Casualty may be unable to speak.
- Casualty may be clutching the upper abdomen and be bent double.
- Possible nausea and vomiting.

AIM
Restore adequate breathing. Seek medical aid only if he or she does not make a full recovery.

TREATMENT
1 Sit the casualty in a relaxed breathing position.

2 If he is unconscious, open his airway and check breathing. Complete the ABC of Resuscitation if required and place him in the Recovery Position (see pp. 14–25).

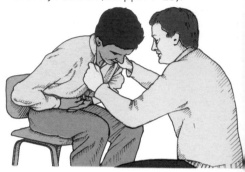

3 Loosen any constricting clothing around his neck, chest and waist.

4 Gently massage his upper abdomen.

HICCUPS

Repeated, noisy intakes of air – hiccups – are caused by involuntary contractions of the diaphragm. Hiccuping attacks generally do not last more than a few minutes and are usually only a minor irritation to the sufferer.

SYMPTOMS & SIGNS
- Frequent noisy intakes of air.

AIM
Break up the sequence of contractions and seek medical aid if the attack is prolonged.

TREATMENT
1 Ask the casualty to sit quietly and hold her breath, or give her long drinks.

2 If this is unsuccessful, place a *paper*, not plastic, bag over the casualty's mouth and nose, and ask her to breathe in and out.

3 If hiccups persist for more than a few hours, seek medical aid.

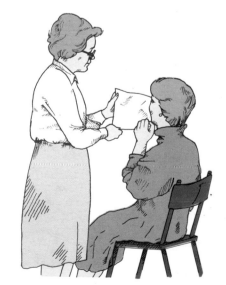

Placing a paper bag over the mouth

WOUNDS & BLEEDING

To operate efficiently the body has to have enough blood circulating at sufficient pressure to reach all the body's tissues all the time. Severe blood loss interferes with the circulation and this can damage the tissues, especially those of the major organs; this may result in the death of the casualty (see *Dangers of Blood Loss*, p.27).

A wound is an abnormal break in the skin or other tissues which allows blood to escape. External wounds are complicated by the fact that germs (bacteria) can enter the tissues and cause infection. Conversely, a casualty may be harbouring an infection in *his* bloodstream which might be transmitted through a break in the unprotected skin of a First Aider. Therefore always wash your hands when possible before and immediately after treating wounds.

TYPES OF WOUND

Wounds are classified as open or closed. Open wounds allow blood to escape from the body. There are several types: incised wounds, lacerated wounds, puncture wounds, grazes, gunshot and contused wounds. Closed wounds allow blood to escape from the circulatory system, but not the body. They may be seen as bruises or collections of blood under the skin or there may be no external evidence.

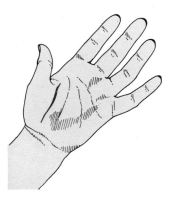

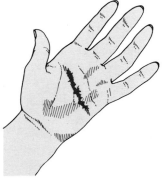

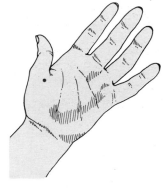

Incised wound
With this type of wound the tissues are cut cleanly by a sharp edge such as a knife, razor or even paper. Such wounds may bleed profusely.

Lacerated wound
The skin may be torn irregularly by contact with barbed wire, machinery or the claws of an animal. These wounds tend to bleed less severely than incised wounds and are frequently contaminated.

Puncture wound
This occurs when the tissues are penetrated by sharp points, e.g., nails, needles, garden forks, railings and teeth, and may result in serious internal injury. If the wound is deep, the risk of infection is high because germs, clothing and dirt may have been carried into it.

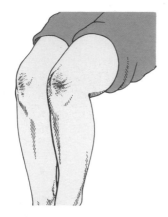
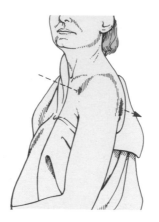
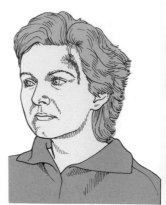

Graze (abrasion)

A graze is usually the result of a sliding fall; superficial layers of skin are scraped off leaving a tender, raw area. These wounds often contain dirt or grit which has become embedded during the injury and may easily become infected (see p.68).

Certain friction burns (see p.135) where the skin has been broken should be treated as grazes.

Gunshot wound

This wound is caused when a missile strikes the body at high speed and can result in serious internal injury. There will be a wound where a missile enters the body and often a much larger exit wound. Internal organs, tissues and blood vessels may be damaged during the missile's passage through the body. In addition to external bleeding, there may be internal bleeding.

Contused wound

This can be caused by a fall or a blow with a blunt object which splits the skin and bruises the surrounding tissues. In a contused wound the risk of damage to underlying structures (e.g., fracture) should be considered.

With a bruise, damaged blood vessels leak blood into the tissues although the skin remains unbroken (see *Bruises*, p.67).

TYPES OF BLEEDING

There are three different types of bleeding: arterial, venous and capillary. Each is named after the type of blood vessel damaged (see *Blood & the Circulation*, p.26). Major arterial bleeding is the most serious and *must* always be treated first (see *Dangers of Blood Loss*, p.27). Capillary bleeding is always present; however, in some wounds arterial and venous bleeding will both be evident.

Arterial bleeding

Blood carried in the arteries is normally fully oxygenated and is bright red. It has just come from the heart so it is under pressure and often spurts from a wound in time with the heartbeat.

Venous bleeding

Normally darker red because it contains less oxygen, venous blood flows at a lower pressure than arterial blood and will not spurt. It may, however, gush profusely if a major vein is ruptured.

Capillary bleeding

This is the most common type of bleeding. It is present in any wound and it may be the only type in minor wounds where blood oozes from the wound.

How the body responds to injury

The natural response of the body to a wound is to restrict local blood flow in order to minimize blood loss. Almost immediately, the ends of the damaged blood vessels contract and nearby vessels become constricted so that local blood flow is reduced. The flow can be further reduced by applying local pressure and elevating the affected part of the body.

In addition, as the blood leaves the damaged vessels it forms a clot. This may be sufficient to plug the hole in the vessel. Once this occurs, repair of the damaged tissues begins. Serum (a watery liquid that separates from the blood after clotting) exudes through the walls of the vessels, carrying antibodies to combat infection and cells which aid the repair process. This causes local swelling. As a result any bandage applied over the wound may become too tight (see p.175).

If the wound is severe and the local mechanisms described are not sufficient to arrest serious bleeding, then all surface vessels constrict. This conserves blood flow to the brain and vital organs. It is this – with accompanying sweating – which gives the skin the pale, clammy appearance of shock (see p.86).

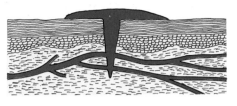

Blood loss from a wound

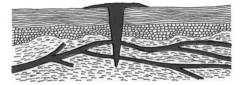

Narrowing of the arteries

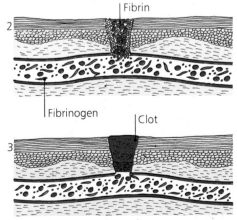

Applying direct pressure

How blood clots are formed

When bleeding occurs, platelets (small particles in the blood) congregate at the site of the injury and help plug the wound (1). Clotting factors are released and a protein present in blood (fibrinogen) is converted into fibrin. This forms a fine mesh across the break, trapping platelets and blood cells (2). The jelly-like mass shrinks as serum oozes out and forms a solid clot over the wound (3).

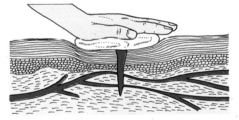

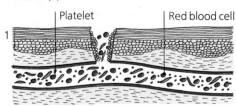

MAJOR EXTERNAL BLEEDING

This occurs most often after a deep incision or laceration in the skin. It is dramatic and may distract you from the priorities of treatment (see pp.31–32).

Always remember that if the casualty is not breathing , begin Artificial Ventilation (see p.18); if he or she is unconscious, maintain an open airway, complete the ABC of Resuscitation (see pp.14–25) and then treat the bleeding. Otherwise, treat the casualty in the position which makes blood control most effective.

Major bleeding must be treated as soon as possible. Follow the order of treatment laid out opposite. Apply direct pressure to the wound and elevate the affected part. This slows down bleeding. Only if direct pressure is not possible or effective and you suspect arterial bleeding, apply indirect pressure (see p.29). Also position the casualty to control blood flow. In some cases you may find that it is only possible to reduce, not actually stop, the flow of blood but this may be enough to preserve life.

Wash your hands with soap and water after treatment.

SYMPTOMS & SIGNS

■ Evidence of major external blood loss.
■ Symptoms and signs of shock (see p.86):
Casualty feels faint and giddy.
Face and lips become pale.
Skin feels cold and clammy.
Pulse becomes faster but weaker.
Casualty may become restless and talkative.
Casualty may complain of thirst.
Breathing may become shallower, sometimes accompanied by yawning and sighing. In more severe cases, deep sighing or gasping (air hunger) may occur.
Vision may be blurred.
Possible unconsciousness.

AIM

Control bleeding and minimize the risk of infection. Arrange urgent removal to hospital.

TREATMENT

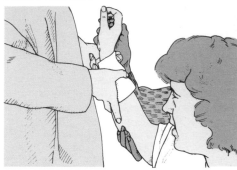

1 Expose the wound and look for foreign bodies (see p.64). Apply direct pressure to control bleeding by pressing with your fingers or palm of your hand over a clean dressing (see p.28). If no dressing is immediately available, use your hands. Alternatively, ask the casualty to use hers. If the wound is gaping, squeezing the edges together may be more effective.

2 Raise and support the part if the wound is on a limb. If you suspect a fracture, see pp.106–123.

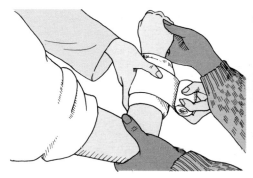

3 Place a sterile or clean dressing and padding over the wound, making sure that it extends well beyond the edges of the wound. Press down firmly and secure with a bandage. Tie bandage firmly enough to control bleeding but not so tight as to cut off circulation (see p.175). Immobilize the injured part (see *Fractures*, pp.106–123).

IF no sterile dressing is available, an improvised dressing can be made from any suitable material (see p.172).

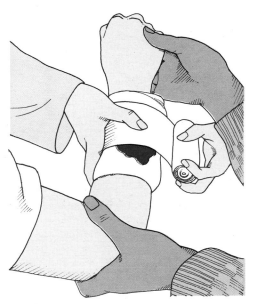

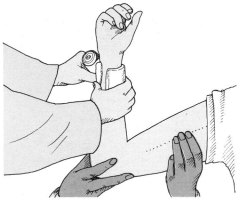

IF the injury is on a limb and direct pressure and elevation is ineffective, apply indirect pressure to the main artery which supplies the limb (see p.29).

DO NOT apply indirect pressure for any longer than 15 minutes (see p.29) nor apply a tourniquet.

4 If bleeding continues, do not remove dressing, but apply further dressings or pads *on top of the original ones* and bandage firmly.

5 To minimize shock, treat as on p.86.

6 Arrange urgent removal to hospital.

AMPUTATIONS

Recent advances in surgery have made the reattachment of amputated limbs, fingers and toes possible. The chances of a good result are greater the sooner the casualty and the severed part are taken to hospital. Always place the severed part in a suitable container to protect it. Inform the ambulance service of an amputation injury immediately so that the hospital can prepare for specialist surgery.

AIM
Control bleeding and arrange urgent removal to hospital with the severed part.

TREATMENT
1 Control bleeding using elevation and direct pressure, see above; take great care not to damage the stump.

2 Place the severed part in a clean plastic bag to keep it clean and prevent it drying out. If possible, put the bag in a container of ice. However, the bag must be wrapped in suitable material to prevent the severed part touching the ice.

NOTE
Mark the package clearly with the casualty's name and the time the amputation occurred.

3 Arrange urgent removal to hospital.

FOREIGN BODIES

Carefully remove any small foreign bodies from the surface of a wound if they can be wiped off easily with a swab or rinsed off with cold water.

If the casualty has a large foreign body embedded in the skin, *never* attempt to remove it. It may be plugging the wound and so restricting bleeding. Moreover, the surrounding tissues may be injured further if it is pulled out.

TREATMENT

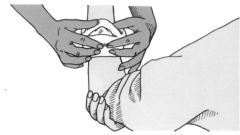

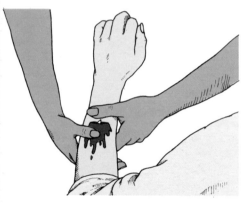

1 To control bleeding, elevate the affected part and apply direct pressure, squeezing the edges of the wound together alongside the foreign body (see p.28). Get the casualty to control bleeding himself if he can do so.

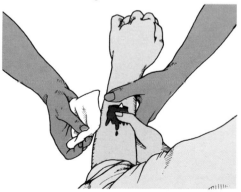

2 Gently place a piece of gauze over and/or around the foreign body.

3 Place crescent-shaped pads of cotton wool or similar material around the wound. If possible, build up the padding until it is high enough to prevent pressure on the object. Secure with a firm bandage.

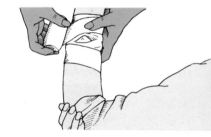

IF it is not possible to build up the padding high enough, leave the foreign body protruding. Secure with a diagonally applied bandage. Make sure the bandage is not over the foreign body.

4 Keeping the injured part elevated, immobilize as far as possible (see *Fractures*, pp.106–123).

5 Arrange urgent removal to hospital, maintaining the treatment position.

IF severe bleeding persists, lay the casualty down and elevate the part. If severe bleeding still continues, use indirect pressure (see p.29).

IF the casualty is impaled on railings or spikes, do not attempt to lift her off, but make her comfortable by supporting the weight of the limbs and trunk. Call an ambulance immediately asking Control to notify the emergency services because cutting tools may be required (see *Calling for Assistance*, p.32).

MINOR EXTERNAL BLEEDING

Many wounds are relatively trivial and involve only slight bleeding. Although blood may ooze from all parts of the wound, it will soon stop of its own accord. A small adhesive dressing is normally all that is necessary, and medical aid need only be sought if there is a serious risk of infection (see p.68).

SYMPTOMS & SIGNS
- Pain at the site of the wound.
- Steady trickle of mixed blood.

AIM
Control bleeding and minimize infection.

TREATMENT

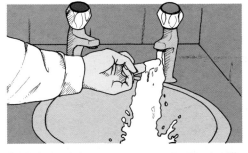

1 If possible wash your hands before dealing with the wound. Then, if the wound is dirty, lightly rinse it with running water, if available, until it is clean.

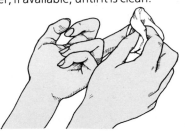

2 Temporarily protect the wound with a sterile swab. Carefully clean the surrounding skin with water and soap if available. Gently wipe away from the wound using each swab once only and taking care not to wipe off any blood clots. Dab gently to dry.

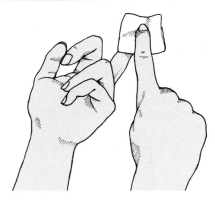

3 If bleeding persists, apply direct pressure (see p.28).

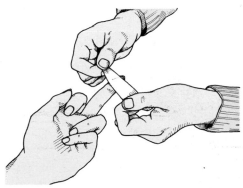

4 Cover a small wound with an appropriate dressing (see p.169–172).

5 Raise and support the injured part.

6 If in any doubt about the injury, seek medical aid.

IF the wound is larger, apply a sterile dressing or gauze and a clean pad, and bandage firmly in position.

INTERNAL BLEEDING

This may occur following an injury such as a fracture, a crush or penetrating injury or because of a medical condition such as a bleeding stomach ulcer. Internal organs, the spleen and liver for example, can be damaged by blows to the body, although there may be no external evidence.

Internal bleeding may be more serious than external bleeding. Although the blood is not actually lost from the body, it is lost from the circulatory system and the vital organs become starved of oxygen (see *Dangers of Blood Loss*, p.27). Blood collecting internally may also cause complications if it presses on vital structures. For example, blood inside the skull can compress the brain causing loss of consciousness; bleeding inside the chest may prevent the lungs expanding.

Blood from internal injuries may collect in one of the body's cavities and remain concealed. Alternatively, it may be revealed by the appearance of discoloration and bruising, or by a flow of blood from one or more of the various openings (orifices) of the body such as the mouth or anus. For example, dark red brown blood resembling coffee grounds may be vomited from the mouth (haematemesis) and is probably caused by a bleeding stomach ulcer. Bright red frothy blood coughed up from the lungs (haemoptysis) may be caused by injury or disease of the lung. Passing blood stained or smoky coloured urine (haematuria) may be the result of bleeding from the bladder or kidney. Blood may appear in the stool with a dark tarry consistency (melaena) indicating bleeding from the upper intestine, or as fresh (bright red) blood indicating bleeding from the lower bowel. Bleeding from the vagina may result from menstrual loss, miscarriage, injury or diseases of the womb.

Always suspect internal bleeding after a violent injury, if there are symptoms and signs of shock without any visible blood loss or if there is any "patterned" bruising corresponding to the seams and/or texture of the casualty's clothing.

SYMPTOMS & SIGNS

These will vary according to the amount of bleeding and the rate at which blood is lost.
■ History of sufficient injury to cause internal bleeding.
■ History of a medical condition which may cause internal bleeding (e.g., ulcer).
■ Pain and tenderness around the affected area; swelling and tension may be felt, as in the thigh.
■ Symptoms and signs of shock (see p.86):
The pulse will increase in rate.
Breathing may be shallow.
Casualty may become restless and talkative.
Casualty may complain of thirst.
■ Blood may appear from one of the body's orifices (see above).

AIM

Arrange urgent removal to hospital because it is not usually possible to control internal bleeding using First Aid.

TREATMENT

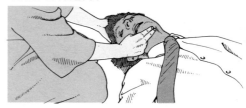

1 Lay the casualty down with his head low and to one side to ensure a good blood supply to his brain. Advise him not to move.

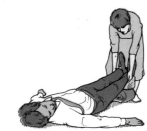

2 If his injuries allow, raise his legs to aid the return of blood flow to the vital organs.

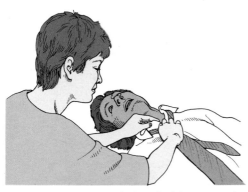

3 Loosen any constricting clothing around his neck, chest and waist.

4 Reassure him and explain the necessity for him to relax.

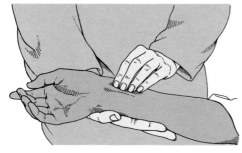

5 Check breathing rate (see p.12), pulse (see p.85) and level of responsiveness (see p.95) at 10-minute intervals. Record these for the doctor.

6 Examine the casualty for other injuries (see pp.33–36) and treat as necessary.

7 If he becomes unconscious, open his airway and check breathing. Complete the ABC of Resuscitation if required and place him in the Recovery Position (see pp.14–25).

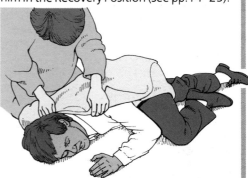

8 Keep the casualty covered and place a blanket underneath him, if possible.

9 Keep a record of any specimen passed or vomited by the casualty. If possible send samples to the hospital with him.

10 Arrange urgent removal to hospital. Transport as a stretcher case, maintaining the treatment postion.

DO NOT give the casualty anything by mouth.

BRUISES

A bruise consists of internal bleeding which seeps through the tissues, and appears as a discoloration under the skin. A heavy fall on fleshy parts of the body, e.g., the buttocks, can result in considerable bruising. A bruise may follow blows, sprains or fractures.

SYMPTOMS & SIGNS
- Pain and swelling in the affected area.
- Bluish-purple discoloration at site of injury.
- Pattern bruising, in which outlines of the casualty's clothing are seen in the bruise. This is a potentially dangerous sign as it may indicate damage to internal organs.

AIM
Slow down blood flow by cooling and gentle compression.

TREATMENT
1 Raise and support the injured part in the position the casualty finds most comfortable.

2 Apply a cold compress to the injured area (see p.173) to restrict bleeding and reduce swelling.

3 If in doubt about the severity of the injury, seek medical aid.

INFECTED WOUNDS

All open wounds will be contaminated by germs which either come from the cause of the injury, from the air or from the First Aider's breath or fingers. Some particles of dirt may be carried away from the damaged tissue by bleeding. Any harmful germs which remain are usually destroyed by the white cells in the blood and the wound then stays clean and healthy.

Normal First Aid for wounds includes prevention of infection. However, any wound which has not begun to heal properly after about 48 hours may be infected because either dirt, dead tissue, foreign bodies and/or bacteria may still be present. If infection develops, it can have serious consequences. It may enter the blood system and subsequently spread to other parts of the body, permanently destroying tissue and occasionally leading to death.

SYMPTOMS & SIGNS
■ Increasing pain and soreness in the wound.
■ Increased swelling and redness of the wound and surrounding parts with a feeling of heat.
■ Pus may ooze from the wound.
■ Fever, sweating, thirst, shivering and lethargy if the infection is severe.
■ Swelling and tenderness in the glands in the neck, armpits or groin.
■ Faint red trails may be seen on the surface of the inside of the arms or legs leading towards lymph glands.

AIM
Seek medical aid.

TREATMENT

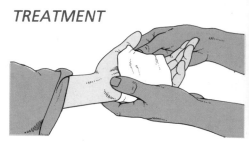

1 Dress wound with a prepared sterile dressing or similar clean, preferably sterile, material and secure with a bandage.

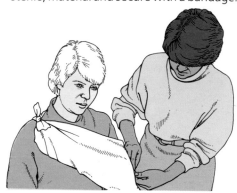

2 Elevate the injured part and immobilize, especially if swollen.

3 Seek medical aid.

TETANUS INFECTION (LOCKJAW)

This particularly dangerous infection results from tetanus germs in a wound which produce a toxic substance. This spreads into the body's nerves, causing severe muscular spasm, particularly in the jaw, hence the name "lockjaw". It is a difficult condition to treat and, if not treated at an early stage, can lead to the death of the casualty.

Every wound carries the risk of tetanus infection, but the disease is preventable by immunization. Everyone should be inoculated against tetanus regularly and you should always ask a wounded casualty how recently inoculation was given. Any casualty with a wound who has never had an anti-tetanus injection or whose last injection was more than five years ago, should be referred for medical advice.

SPECIAL FORMS OF BLEEDING

There are a number of wounds and special forms of bleeding where the treatment does not follow the general rules of direct and indirect pressure and/or position of the injured part. Treatment for these wounds is described on the following pages.

SCALP WOUNDS

Injuries to the scalp most often occur during falls and are particularly common amongst the elderly, ill or intoxicated. Other causes include road traffic accidents, fights, sporting accidents, and falling debris.

Scalp wounds can bleed profusely due to the rich supply of blood to the scalp and because the skin covering the skull is normally stretched. When damaged the skin splits open, leaving a gaping wound. This bleeding may appear more alarming than it really is, but the casualty may also have a skull fracture.

SYMPTOMS & SIGNS
■ Pain, tenderness and bleeding of the scalp. Possible lifted flap of scalp.
■ Swelling around the wound.
■ Possible symptoms and signs of skull fracture (see p.100).
■ Signs of brain damage may be evident (see *Concussion* and *Compression*, pp.98–99).
■ Unconsciousness may develop.

AIM
Control bleeding as soon as possible. Arrange removal to hospital as *all* head injuries should be examined by a doctor.

TREATMENT

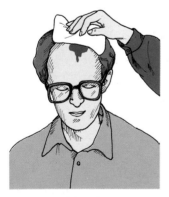

NOTE
The head bandage does not provide adequate pressure for the control of severe bleeding.

1 Control the bleeding using direct pressure (p.28). Cover the wound with a sterile or clean dressing or a pad of clean material (these should be larger than the wound). Retain with a bandage (see p.181).

2 If the casualty is conscious, carefully and gently lay him down with his head and shoulders slightly raised.

3 Check the casualty's breathing rate (see p.12), pulse (see p.85) and level of responsiveness (see p.95) at 10-minute intervals.

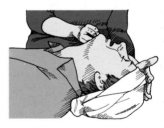

4 If the casualty becomes unconscious, open his airway and check breathing. Complete the ABC of Resuscitation if required and place him in the Recovery Postion with the injured side uppermost (see pp.14–25).

5 Arrange urgent removal to hospital. Transport the casualty as a stretcher case, maintaining the treatment position.

BLEEDING FROM THE EAR

Bleeding from inside the ear canal differs from that found in external ear wounds. It generally occurs when an eardrum ruptures or when a skull fracture is present (see p.100). A perforated eardrum can result from pushing an object into the ear (see p.160), falling while water-skiing, diving, or being too near an explosion.

Skull fractures are more serious and should be suspected if blood or clear, watery cerebro-spinal fluid mixed with blood is issuing from the ear.

SYMPTOMS & SIGNS

If from the eardrum
- Possible pain inside the ear.
- Deafness.
- Moderate flow of blood from the ear.

If from within the skull
- History indicating possible skull fracture (see p.100) or other head injury (see p.98).
- Casualty complains of a headache.
- Small amounts of blood mixed with clear, watery cerebro-spinal fluid may be coming from the ear.
- Possible unconsciousness.

AIM

Arrange removal to hospital. If skull fracture is suspected, pay particular attention to the level of responsiveness (see p.95).

TREATMENT

1 Place the conscious casualty in a half-sitting position with his head inclined towards the injured side so that blood or fluid can drain.

2 Cover the ear with a sterile dressing or similar clean, preferably sterile, material. Secure it very lightly with a bandage or adhesive strapping.

> **DO NOT** plug the ear or try to stop the flow from the ear; pressure may build up inside the middle ear.

3 Check breathing rate (see p.12), pulse (see p.85) and level of responsiveness (see p.95) at 10-minute intervals.

4 To minimize shock, treat as on p.86.

5 If the casualty becomes unconscious, open his airway and check breathing. Complete the ABC of Resuscitation if required and place him in the Recovery Position (see pp.14–25); his head should lie on the injured side to allow fluid to drain.

6 Arrange removal to hospital. Transport as a stretcher case, maintaining the treatment position.

NOSE-BLEEDS

This is a common condition usually due to bleeding from the blood vessels inside the nostrils. It may occur after a blow to the nose or be the result of sneezing, picking or blowing the nose. However, watery-looking, blood-stained fluid issuing from the nose may be a sign of a fractured skull (see p.100).

Nose-bleeds can cause considerable loss of blood and may also cause the casualty to swallow or inhale a great deal of blood. This may cause vomiting or affect breathing.

SYMPTOMS & SIGNS
■ Moderate flow of blood from nose.
■ If skull fracture is present, there may be a mixture of blood and clear, watery cerebro-spinal fluid.

AIM
Safeguard the breathing by preventing inhalation of blood, and control bleeding.

TREATMENT
1 Sit the casualty down with her head well forward and loosen any tight clothing around her neck and chest.

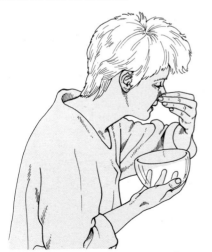

2 Advise her to breathe through her mouth and to pinch the soft part of her nose. (Be prepared to take over if it is tiring for her).

3 Forbid speech, swallowing, coughing, spitting or sniffing. Allow her to dribble, and mop it up.

4 Release the pressure after 10 minutes. If the bleeding has not stopped, continue treatment for further periods of 10 minutes as necessary.

DO NOT let the casualty raise her head.

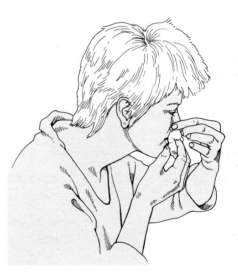

5 While the head is still forward, if possible get the casualty gently to clean around the nose and mouth using a swab or clean dressing soaked in luke-warm water. Do not plug the nose.

6 When the bleeding stops, tell the casualty to avoid exertion and not to blow her nose for at least four hours so as not to disturb the clot.

7 If after 30 minutes the bleeding persists or recurs, seek medical aid.

71

BLEEDING FROM THE MOUTH

Cuts in the tongue, lips or lining of the mouth range from trivial injuries to larger wounds. They are usually caused by the casualty's teeth during falls or a blow to the face. Bleeding may be severe.

Bleeding can also occur from the tooth socket after accidental loss of a tooth or some time after a dental extraction. Laceration of the gums may occur in association with a fracture of the jaw.

SYMPTOMS & SIGNS

■ Bleeding in or around the mouth or from a tooth socket.
■ Pain in the affected area.

AIM

Safeguard the airway by preventing the inhalation of blood, and control bleeding.

TREATMENT

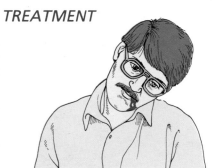

1 Ask the casualty to sit down with his head forward and inclined towards the injured side.

2 To control bleeding, place a clean dressing over any external wound and tell the casualty to apply direct pressure by squeezing it between his thumb and finger. If a tooth socket is bleeding, place a thick pad of gauze or clean coth across, not in, the socket.

NOTE
This pad must be thick enough to prevent teeth meeting when the casualty bites.

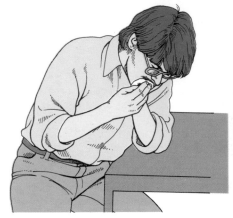

3 The casualty should maintain pressure on the dressing or pad for 10–20 minutes, supporting his chin on his hand.

4 Allow him to dribble out any blood in his mouth while maintaining pressure; swallowed blood can cause vomiting.

5 If bleeding persists after 10–20 minutes, carefully remove dressing or pad, disturbing the clot as little as possible. Renew dressing or pad and continue pressure for a further 10 minutes.

NOTE
This is an exception to the rule that you leave the first dressing in place when you apply a further dressing.

DO NOT wash out the mouth as this may disturb the clot. Advise the casualty to avoid all hot drinks for 12 hours.

6 If the bleeding persists or recurs, seek medical or dental aid.

7 If the casualty has lost a tooth and it can be found, place it in a clean container, seek dental aid as soon as possible and send the tooth with the casualty.

EYE WOUNDS

All eye injuries are potentially serious. Even superficial grazes can lead to scarring of the surface of the eye (cornea) or infection, with possible deterioration of eyesight and even permanent blindness.

The eye can be cut or bruised by direct blows, broken spectacles, or sharp, chipped fragments of metallic materials, grit or glass which fly into it.

For treatment of foreign bodies in the eye, see p.159.

SYMPTOMS & SIGNS
■ Partial or total loss of vision of the affected eye, even with no visible injury.
■ Painful, bloodshot eye, possibly with a visible wound of eyeball or eyelid.
■ Loss of blood or clear fluid from the eye wound, possibly with flattening of the normal round contour of the eyeball as the contents leak.

AIM
Protect the eye by preventing movement and seek medical aid.

TREATMENT
1 Lay the casualty down on his back. Support his head and keep it as still as possible.

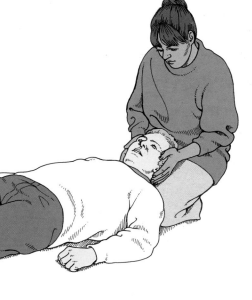

DO NOT attempt to remove embedded foreign bodies.

2 Ask the casualty to close his injured eye and gently cover it with an eyepad or a sterile dressing. Secure it with a bandage or adhesive plaster.

3 Advise the casualty to keep his sound eye still because movement will cause the injured eye to move. If necessary, bandage both eyes to prevent unnecessary movement. Reassure the casualty before blindfolding.

4 Arrange removal to hospital, maintaining the treatment position.

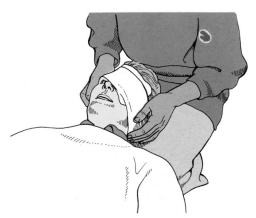

WOUNDS TO THE PALM OF THE HAND

Wounds in the palm can occur when a person handles broken glass or sharp tools or falls on to sharp objects. Such wounds may bleed profusely and can be accompanied by fractures. If the wound is deep, the nerves and tendons in the hand may be damaged.

SYMPTOMS & SIGNS
■ Pain at the site of the wound.
■ Bleeding which may be profuse.
■ Loss of sensation and movement in the fingers and hand if the underlying nerves and tendons are severed.

AIM
Control bleeding and arrange urgent removal to hospital *without* attempting to remove any embedded foreign bodies.

TREATMENT

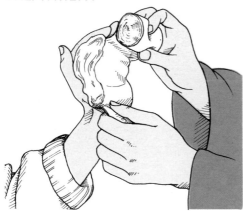

1 To control bleeding, place a sterile dressing or gauze and a clean pad over the wound and apply direct pressure with your fingers or thumbs (see p.28) or by casualty if able.

IF no dressing or pad is available, use an improvised dressing (see p.172).

2 Elevate the injured arm above the level of the heart.

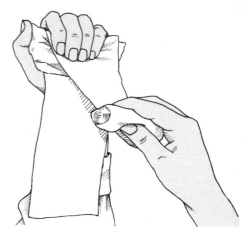

3 Ask the casualty to maintain pressure by clenching her fist over the dressing or pad.

IF the casualty cannot do this, tell her to grasp the fist of her injured hand with her other hand.

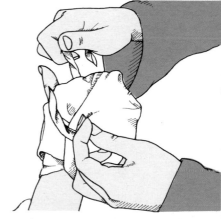

4 Bandage the fist firmly, using the loose ends of the dressing or a folded triangular bandage. Tie off firmly across the bent fingers to maintain pressure.

5 Support the arm in an elevation sling (see p.179) and arrange removal to hospital.

BLEEDING VARICOSE VEINS

The veins in the legs contain valves to keep the blood flowing back to the heart. When these valves deteriorate, they leak backwards and the back pressure of the blood causes the veins to become swollen and "knobbly" or "varicose". Such veins can be burst by quite gentle knocks and they bleed severely. If such bleeding is not controlled immediately the condition can be fatal.

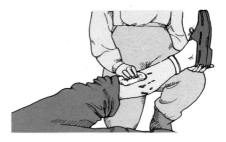

SYMPTOMS & SIGNS

■ Severe external bleeding; blood will be dark red.
■ Symptoms and signs of shock (see p.86).
■ Unconsciousness may develop.

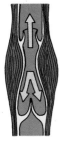
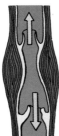

A damaged valve (right) will prevent the correct blood flow (left)

AIM

Control bleeding by elevation and direct pressure. Arrange urgent removal to hospital.

TREATMENT

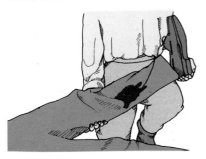

1 Lay the casualty on his back and raise the injured leg as high as possible.

2 Expose the wound and apply direct pressure by pressing with your fingers or palm of your hand over a dressing (p.28).

3 Remove any constricting clothing such as elastic-topped or support stockings, garters or tights which may be impeding blood flow back to the heart.

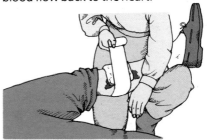

4 Place a soft pad over the dressing large enough to exert pressure on the whole area around the bleeding varicose vein. Tie a bandage firmly enough to control bleeding but not so tight as to cut off circulation (see p.175).

IF no sterile dressing is available, use an improvised dressing (see p.172).

IF bleeding does not stop and bandages are soaked with blood, apply further padding and bandages on top of the original ones.

5 Keep the leg raised and supported.

6 To minimize shock, treat as on p.86.

7 Arrange urgent removal to hospital, maintaining the treatment postion.

PENETRATING CHEST WOUNDS

The ribcage protects not only the heart, lungs and major blood vessels in the chest cavity above the diaphragm, but also the liver and spleen below the diaphragm in the upper abdominal cavity.

A wound to the front or back of the chest which penetrates into the chest allows air to enter the space occupied by the lungs, thus interfering with breathing.

In these injuries, the lung on the affected side collapses, even if it is not punctured. Air in the chest cavity impairs the action of the sound lung and, sometimes, of the heart. The amount of oxygen reaching the blood stream may be insufficient and asphyxia may result (see p.42).

A wound to the front or back of the lower chest may penetrate into the abdominal cavity and give rise to severe internal bleeding.

SYMPTOMS & SIGNS

- Casualty may have pain in the chest.
- May have an acute sense of alarm.
- Difficulty in breathing; breaths are shallow due to air in the chest cavity.
- Blueness of the mouth, nailbeds and skin (cyanosis) indicating the onset of significant asphyxia.
- Bright red, frothy blood may be coughed up
- The sound of air being sucked into the chest may be heard when the casualty is breathing in.
- Blood-stained liquid bubbling from the chest wound during breathing out.
- Symptoms and signs of shock (see p.86).

AIM

Ease breathing by immediately sealing the wound. Arrange urgent removal to hospital.

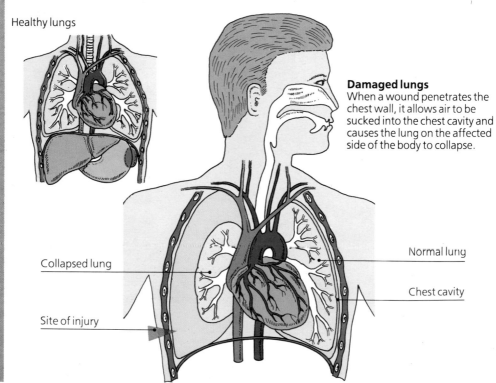

Healthy lungs

Damaged lungs
When a wound penetrates the chest wall, it allows air to be sucked into the chest cavity and causes the lung on the affected side of the body to collapse.

Collapsed lung

Normal lung

Chest cavity

Site of injury

TREATMENT

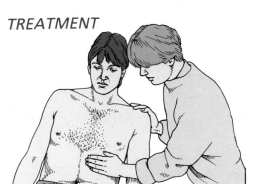

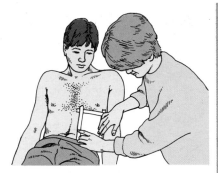

1 Immediately seal the open wound with your palm or the casualty's if possible.

5 If possible, form an airtight seal by covering the dressing with a plastic sheet or metal foil. Secure and seal the edges of the dressing with layers of adhesive tape, strapping and/or bandage.

6 Support the arm on the injured side in an elevation sling (see p.179) and make the casualty as comfortable as possible.

7 Check breathing rate (see p.12), pulse (see p.85) and level of responsiveness (see p.95) at 10-minute intervals. Look for evidence of internal bleeding (see p.66).

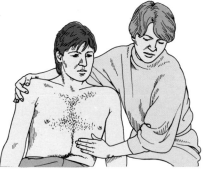

2 Place the casualty in a half-sitting position with his head and shoulders supported; turn the body towards the injured side so the sound lung is uppermost.

3 Reassure the casualty.

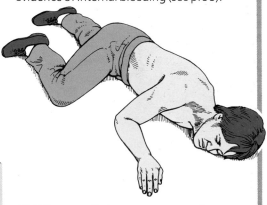

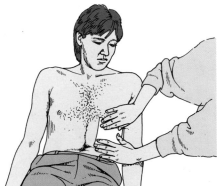

8 If the casualty becomes unconscious, open his airway and check breathing. Complete the ABC of Resuscitation if required and place him in the Recovery Position with his uninjured side uppermost (see pp.14–25).

9 Arrange urgent removal to hospital. Transport as a stretcher case, maintaining the treatment position.

4 Gently cover the wounds with a sterile dressing as soon as possible.

IF a foreign body is present, see p.64.

ABDOMINAL WOUNDS

Wounds of the abdominal wall may be caused by sharp instruments or by missiles. A deep wound of the abdominal wall is serious not only because of the external bleeding, but also because the underlying organs may have been punctured or lacerated, leading to severe internal bleeding and possible infection. Part of the intestine may also be protruding from the wound.

SYMPTOMS & SIGNS
■ General abdominal pain.
■ Bleeding and associated wounds (which may only be a small puncture) in the abdominal area.
■ Part of the intestine may be visible in, or protruding from, the wound.
■ Casualty may be vomiting.
■ Symptoms and signs of shock (see p.86).

AIM
Protect wound to minimize infection, and arrange urgent removal to hospital.

TREATMENT

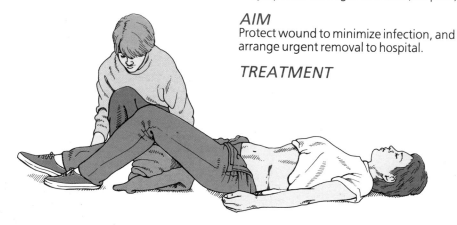

1 Lay the casualty on her back with her knees bent up to prevent the wound gaping and to reduce strain on the injured area. Support her knees.

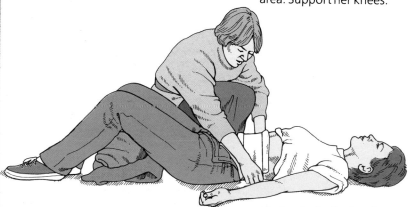

2 Apply sterile dressing or gauze and a clean pad over the wound and secure with a bandage or adhesive strapping.

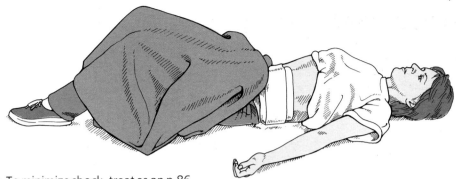

3 To minimize shock, treat as on p.86.

DO NOT remove protruding objects or give the casualty anything by mouth.

4 Check breathing rate (see p.12) and pulse (see p.85) at 10-minute intervals. Look for evidence of internal bleeding (see p.66).

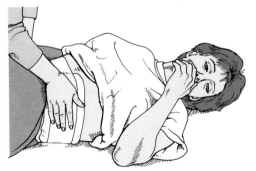

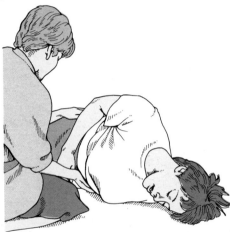

6 If she becomes unconscious, open her airway and check breathing. Complete the ABC of Resuscitation if required, and support her abdomen when placing her in the Recovery Position (see pp.14–25).

5 If the casualty coughs or vomits, support her abdomen by pressing gently on the dressing to prevent protrusion of the intestines from the wound.

7 Arrange urgent removal to hospital. Transport as a stretcher case, maintaining the treatment position.

IF PART OF THE INTESTINE PROTRUDES FROM THE WOUND

DO NOT touch the protruding intestines.

1 Cover with a sterile dressing or clean cloth secured with a bandage.

2 If the casualty coughs or vomits, support the wound as in step 5.

3 Position and treat the casualty as above.

VAGINAL BLEEDING

This can be severe menstrual bleeding or the result of a miscarriage, internal injury or sexual assault. The history of the condition is essential to the diagnosis of the emergency. If you suspect a miscarriage, treat as described on p.207.

Heavy menstrual bleeding or miscarriage may also be accompanied by severe cramps. These normally occur at the beginning of the period but may last for several days.

SYMPTOMS & SIGNS

■ Moderate to severe bleeding from the vagina.
■ Symptoms and signs of shock may be present (see p.86).
■ Cramp-like pains in the lower abdomen or pelvic area.

AIM

Reassure the casualty and if in doubt about the severity of the bleeding, arrange removal to hospital.

TREATMENT

1 If possible, remove the woman to a place which has some privacy or arrange for screening. Give her a sanitary dressing, if available, or a clean towel to place over the entrance of the vagina.

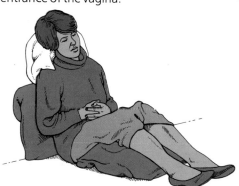

2 Lay the woman down with her head and shoulders raised and her knees bent, supported on a blanket. (This will relax the abdominal muscles.)

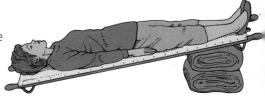

3 If the pains are severe, and obviously due to menstruation, let her take one or two of her own pain-killing tablets or those made specifically for the relief of menstrual cramps if available.

4 If bleeding continues and is severe, minimize shock by treating as on p.86. Arrange urgent removal to hospital, maintaining the treatment position.

CRUSH INJURIES

These injuries commonly occur in earthquakes, bomb incidents, mining accidents and demolition work. Prolonged crushing of a mass of muscles, e.g., in the thigh, leads to shock because of the blood loss into the tissues after the casualty has been freed. Toxic substances released by the damaged muscles are introduced into the casualty's circulation and may lead to kidney failure. This sequence is known as "the crush syndrome".

Because of the danger of kidney failure, in all cases where a casualty has been trapped for longer than one hour, call the emergency services immediately and do not attempt to release him or her.

SYMPTOMS & SIGNS
- Crushed limb may be tingling or numb.
- Swollen and hard tissue around injured part because serum (see p.61) has poured into the area.
- Bruising and formation of blisters at the site of injury.
- Crushed or trapped limb will be cool, pale and pulseless if arteries are compressed.
- Symptoms and signs of fracture (see p.108).
- Symptoms and signs of shock (see p.86).

AIM
Prevent damage to the kidneys. Arrange urgent medical assistance if the casualty has been trapped for more than one hour.

TREATMENT

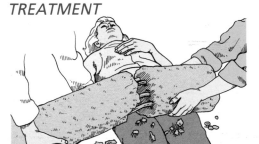

2 Elevate the limb if the injuries allow you to do so.

3 Control any bleeding and treat any wounds.

4 Immobilize any fractures if present (see pp.106–123).

5 Position as for treatment of shock (see p.86) and remove to hospital if necessary.

IF TRAPPED FOR LESS THAN ONE HOUR

1 Release the casualty as quickly as possible.

NOTE
Record time of release and duration of crushing.

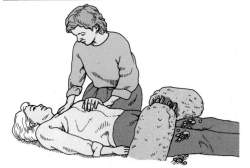

IF TRAPPED FOR MORE THAN ONE HOUR

DO NOT attempt to release the casualty.

1 Reassure and make her as comfortable as the circumstances permit.

2 Call for medical assistance and emergency services.

ANIMAL BITES

Germs are harboured in the mouths of all animals. Most animals have sharp, pointed teeth. Because of this, their bites often leave deep puncture wounds and germs may be injected deep into the tissues. Human bites are worse because they crush the tissues.

Any bite causing a break in the skin needs prompt attention to prevent infection. It may be complicated by tetanus (see p.68) and in some countries rabies (see below). Savaging by a dog may also result in multiple lacerations of the skin and muscles.

SYMPTOMS & SIGNS
■ One or more small puncture wounds in the pattern of the teeth.
■ A number of lacerations indicating a tearing bite.
■ Bleeding can be severe or may be slight, depending on the extent of the injury.

AIM
Treat the wound and seek medical aid: arrange urgent removal to hospital if the wound is serious. Report dog bites to the police.

TREATMENT

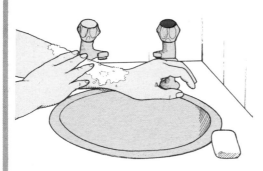 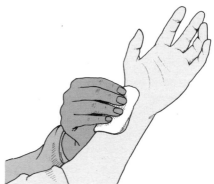

FOR SUPERFICIAL BITES
1 Wash the wound thoroughly with soapy water for five minutes. Dry it and cover with a sterile dressing.

2 Seek medical aid.

FOR SERIOUS WOUNDS
1 Control any serious bleeding with direct pressure and elevation (see p.28).

2 Cover with a sterile dressing and bandage securely.

3 Arrange removal of the casualty to hospital.

RABIES

This is a potentially fatal condition spread by the saliva of infected animals. Although not currently found in the United Kingdom, rabies is endemic in many countries. Therefore, if an animal bite is sustained in a foreign country or if you suspect an infected animal may have been smuggled into the United Kingdom, you *must* make sure that the casualty has a course of injections.

To confirm or exclude a rabies infection, the animal must be examined medically. If possible, attempt to isolate the animal, *without* endangering yourself. If the animal escapes, notify the police immediately.

SNAKE BITES

The only poisonous snake native to the United Kingdom is the adder. However, there are many poisonous snakes kept as pets, some of which may escape or attack their owners. In addition to the injuries produced by a bite, fright resulting in severe shock may also be evident. Contrary to popular belief, snake bites are only rarely fatal.

In countries where there are numerous dangerous snakes, it is important to identify the snake so that appropriate anti-venom serum can be administered. Therefore, record its description (colour and markings are the best guide) or if it has been captured or killed, keep it.

SYMPTOMS & SIGNS
■ Casualty may experience disturbed vision.
■ Casualty may feel nauseated or already be vomiting.
■ One or two small puncture wounds with sharp pain and local swelling.
■ Breathing may become difficult or fail altogether.
■ Symptoms and signs of shock (see p.86).
■ Salivation and sweating may appear in advanced stages of venom reaction.

AIM
Reassure the casualty, prevent absorption of venom, and arrange urgent removal to hospital.

TREATMENT

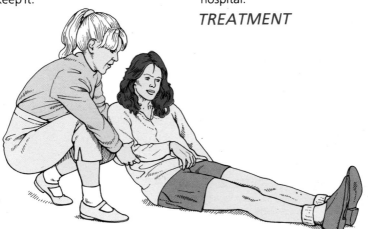

1 Lay the casualty down and advise her not to move.

2 Immobilize the affected part, but do not elevate it.

3 Wash the wound thoroughly with soap and water, if available.

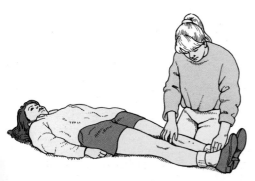

4 If the casualty becomes unconscious, open her airway and check breathing. Complete the ABC of Resuscitation if required and place her in the Recovery Postion (see pp.14–25).

5 Arrange removal to hospital. If possible take the snake in a safe container.

CIRCULATORY DISORDERS

Blood is pumped around the body by the heart through blood vessels to the tissues and cells of the body, before returning via the heart to the lungs where it is re-oxygenated (see *Blood & the Circulation*, pp.26–27).

There are several factors which affect circulation:

■ The volume and quality of the blood in the system.

■ The pressure at which the blood is circulated.

■ The condition of the heart and blood vessels through which the blood flows. Changes in any of these factors can lead to circulatory disorders.

The composition of the blood is vital to the health of the tissues. Normal blood consists of a transparent yellow fluid called plasma in which the red cells, white cells and platelets are suspended. The coloured pigment in the red cells (haemoglobin) carries oxygen to the tissues. The white cells help protect the body against infection. The platelets, along with clotting factors and fibrinogen, assist the blood to clot (see p.61).

The average adult has six litres (10 pints) of blood circulating in the body. Normal blood pressure is the pumping force of the heart required to ensure blood reaches all the tissues. It depends on the strength of the heartbeat and the condition of the blood vessels. If it is too low, e.g., due to loss of blood volume, the vital organs will be unable to function properly, and the symptoms and signs of shock may develop (see p.86). If the blood pressure is continually too high (common as age increases), and perhaps in association with hardening of the arteries, rupture of a blood vessel may occur, giving rise to internal bleeding (e.g., cerebral haemorrhage, a form of stroke).

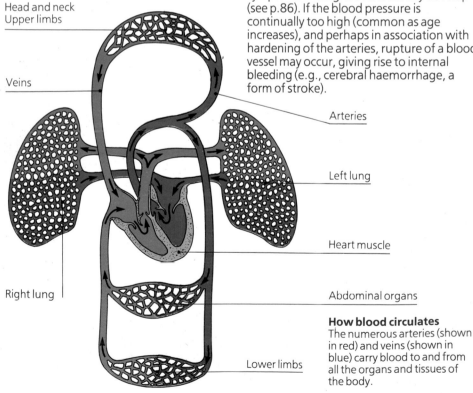

Head and neck
Upper limbs

Veins

Arteries

Left lung

Heart muscle

Right lung

Abdominal organs

Lower limbs

How blood circulates
The numerous arteries (shown in red) and veins (shown in blue) carry blood to and from all the organs and tissues of the body.

Poor blood circulation, possibly aggravated by the slowing down process of advancing years, can contribute to the formation of a clot (thrombus), as can narrowed blood vessels, which may also have "fatty" deposits on their walls. A clot carried up into the artery of the brain can cause stroke (cerebral embolism); a clot carried to the lungs can affect the oxygenation process (pulmonary embolism).

The heart muscle (myocardium) contracts and relaxes in the same way as other muscles and it has its own separate blood supply – the coronary arteries. However, unlike other muscles, it must function continuously in order to sustain all the other organs of the body by supplying them with blood.

The coronary arteries, like all other arteries, can become narrowed so that the amount of blood able to pass through

them to the heart muscle is reduced, causing pain (angina pectoris). A clot may form in the coronary arteries and cause a heart attack (coronary thrombosis/myocardial infarction).

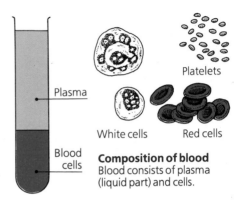

Plasma

Platelets

White cells   Red cells

Blood cells

Composition of blood
Blood consists of plasma (liquid part) and cells.

THE PULSE

This is the wave of pressure which passes along the arteries, indicating the pumping action of the heart. It can be felt where an artery is close to the surface of the body and can be pressed against a bone.

The most useful pulse, the carotid pulse, can be felt just below the angle of the jaw in the hollow between the voice box and adjoining muscle (see p.17). However, unless cardiac arrest is suspected, the pulse is usually taken at the wrist.

To take the radial pulse, place the pads of three fingertips in the hollow immediately above the creases in front of the wrist in line with the base of the thumb, and press lightly against the underlying bone. (Do not use your thumb because it has a pulse of is own.) To take the pulse, count the number of beats in a minute.

The three things to check and record are the rate, strength (strong or weak), and rhythm (regular or irregular). The normal pulse rate in an adult can vary between 60 and 80 beats per minute. It increases during stress, exercise, some illnesses,

while taking alcohol or as a result of injury. The pulse rate in some athletes may be normally slower, and in some young babies, normally faster.

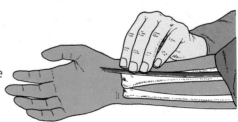

Checking the radial pulse

NOTE
In babies and young children, the carotid or radial pulse may be difficult to find. In these circumstances, the brachial pulse may be used (see p.23).

SHOCK

This is a manifestation of changes in which the circulation fails because either the pressure or volume of circulating blood has fallen to a dangerous level (see pp.27 and 28). This is because the blood flowing to the vital organs is insufficient to keep them supplied with oxygen and functioning. It is a serious condition which can prove fatal.

There are many possible causes of shock and they fall into two main groups. Firstly, the heart pump may fail so that the pressure of the circulating blood becomes weak. Examples of this group include the effects of electrocution, and blockages in the coronary blood vessels which supply the heart muscle. Secondly, the volume of blood in circulation around the body may become reduced, e.g., in external or internal bleeding. In burns, vomiting or diarrhoea, the fluid part of the blood may be reduced so that the volume shrinks and shock occurs.

The body reacts to shock by diverting available blood to the vital organs (e.g., brain, heart and kidneys) away from less important tissues (e.g., skin).

Pain, fear or an upright posture can aggravate the effect of shock.

SYMPTOMS & SIGNS

As the casualty's condition deteriorates, the symptoms and signs will become more pronounced.
■ Casualty becomes pale or grey in colour (most obvious inside the lips).
■ Skin is cold and moist with sweat.
■ Casualty may feel weak, faint or giddy.
■ The pulse becomes weak and rapid.
■ Breathing is shallow and fast.
■ Casualty may become anxious or restless, yawn or gasp (air hunger).
■ Casualty may complain of thirst.
■ Casualty may feel sick and may vomit.
■ Possible unconsciousness.

AIM

Improve blood supply to brain, heart and lungs, and arrange urgent removal to hospital.

TREATMENT

DO NOT move the casualty unnecessarily.

1 Treat any cause you can remedy, e.g., external bleeding. Move the casualty as little as possible and reassure him.

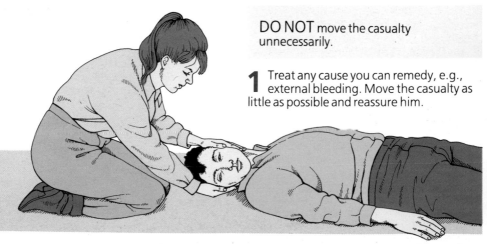

2 Lay him down, keeping his head low and to one side to lessen the dangers of vomiting.

3 Raise his legs and rest them on folded clothes or other suitable props. If you suspect a leg fracture, see pp.116–120.

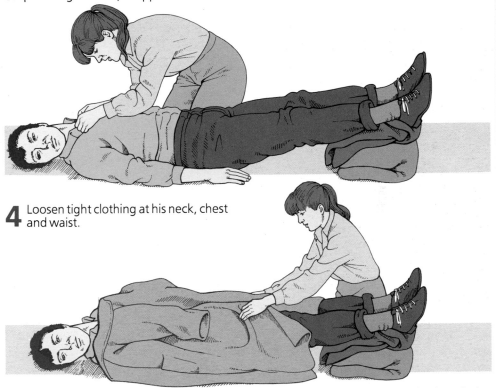

4 Loosen tight clothing at his neck, chest and waist.

5 Shelter him from extremes of temperature. Keep him comfortable, wrapping a blanket, rug or coat around him if necessary. Moisten his lips with water but do not give him anything to drink.

6 Treat any other injuries.

7 Check breathing rate (see p.12), pulse (see p.85) and level of responsiveness (see p.95) at 10-minute intervals.

8 If breathing becomes difficult or vomiting likely, place him in the Recovery Position (see p.24).

9 If he becomes unconscious, open his airway and check breathing. Complete the ABC of Resuscitation if required and place the casualty in the Recovery Position (see pp.14–25).

10 Arrange urgent removal to hospital, maintaining the treatment position (raise foot of stretcher).

NOTE
Reassure the casualty and stay with him at all times.

DO NOT give him anything to eat or drink – it will delay the subsequent administration of an anaesthetic.

DO NOT apply hot-water bottles – this will increase the blood flow to the skin and take it away from the vital organs.

DO NOT allow the casualty to smoke.

FAINTING

A faint is a brief loss of consciousness of no more than momentary duration caused by a temporary reduction in the flow of blood to the brain. Recovery is usually rapid and complete.

It may be a nervous reaction to pain or fright; or the result of an emotional upset, exhaustion or lack of food. It is, however, more common after long periods of physical inactivity, especially in warm atmospheres, where lack of muscular activity causes a large volume of blood to collect in the lower part of the body and legs. This reduces the amount of blood available to the circulation, e.g., as in a soldier standing on parade.

SYMPTOMS & SIGNS
- Pulse will be slow at first (this is an important clue) and weak.
- Casualty may be very pale.

AIM
Position the casualty so that gravity helps increase the flow of blood to the brain.

PREVENTION
IF the casualty is on parade or standing in a crowd, advise him or her to flex the leg muscles and toes to aid circulation.

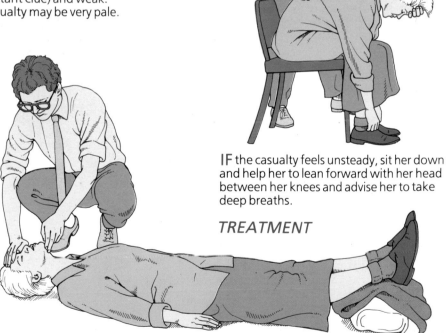

IF the casualty feels unsteady, sit her down and help her to lean forward with her head between her knees and advise her to take deep breaths.

TREATMENT

1 When a casualty faints, lay her down with her legs raised, and maintain an open airway.

2 Loosen any tight clothing at her neck, chest and waist, to assist circulation and breathing.

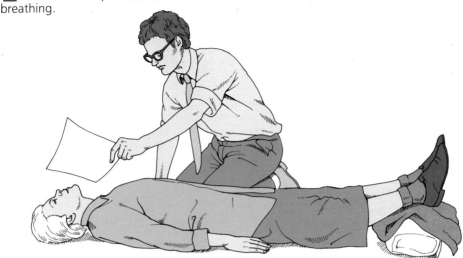

3 Make sure that the casualty has plenty of fresh air: place her in a current of fresh air and fan air on to her face. If necessary, place her in the shade.

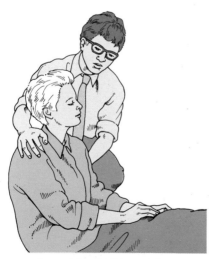

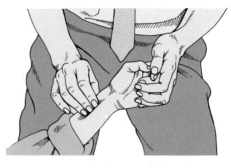

6 Check breathing rate (see p.12), pulse (see p.85), and level of responsiveness (see p.95) until fully recovered.

IF the casualty does not begin to regain consciousness rapidly, open her airway and check breathing. Complete the ABC of Resuscitation if required and place her in the Recovery Position (see pp.14–25). Summon medical aid, and seek other causes for unconsciousness (see pp.37–38).

4 Reassure her whilst she is regaining consciousness; gradually raise her to a sitting position.

5 Check for and treat any injury that she may have sustained on falling.

DO NOT give the casualty anything by mouth until she is fully conscious.

DO NOT give the casualty any alcohol.

HEART DISORDERS

The commonest forms of heart disorder are angina pectoris, coronary obstruction or thrombosis, and cardiac arrest. Sudden interference with the normal action of the heart will have serious consequences. Interference can occur if a blood clot blocks a coronary artery (coronary obstruction/thrombosis), preventing blood reaching the heart muscle, so causing death of an area of the muscle wall (myocardial infarction). This may cause the heart to stop (cardiac arrest).

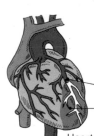

Blocked artery causing possible coronary obstruction, coronary thrombosis or myocardial infarction

Clot (thrombus)

Damaged area (infarct)

Heart muscle (myocardium)

ANGINA PECTORIS

Severe pains in the chest occur when the coronary arteries, which supply blood to the heart, become too narrow for sufficient oxygenated blood to reach the muscles of the heart.

This condition is common in the elderly and is usually brought on by over-exertion during exercise, and sometimes by excitement. Normally these attacks only last a few minutes and the pain stops if the casualty rests.

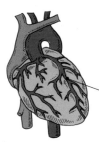

"Narrowed" artery causing reduced blood supply to muscle resulting in possible angina pectoris

"Narrowed" artery

SYMPTOMS & SIGNS

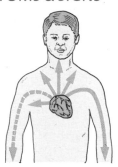

- Pain in chest often spreading down the left shoulder to arm and fingers. (It may also spread to the casualty's throat and jaw and across to the other arm.)
- Skin may be ashen and lips may be blue.
- Casualty may be short of breath.
- General weakness.

AIM

Place the casualty in a resting position in which the heart is able to work most effectively.

TREATMENT

1 Help the casualty to sit down. Support him by placing a blanket or jacket behind him, and padding under the knees.

2 Reassure him and advise to rest. Loosen clothing around his neck, chest and waist.

3 If symptoms persist, arrange removal to hospital.

NOTE

Many people who suffer from angina pectoris carry special medicine with them for the prevention or relief of an attack, and this may be taken.

HEART ATTACK

This term covers coronary thrombosis, coronary obstruction, myocardial infarction and other forms of heart disease.

SYMPTOMS & SIGNS

- Sudden crushing, vice-like pain in the centre of the chest (sometimes described as severe indigestion) which may spread to the arms, throat, jaw, abdomen or back, and does not subside with rest.
- Sudden dizziness or giddiness causing the casualty to sit down or lean against a wall.
- Skin may be ashen; lips and extremities may become blue (cyanosis).
- Profuse sweating may develop.
- Breathlessness can occur.
- Fast pulse, which becomes weaker and may become irregular.
- Symptoms and signs of shock (see p.86).
- Unconsciousness may develop.
- Breathing and heartbeat may stop.

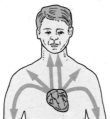

AIM

Minimize the work of the heart and obtain medical aid. Arrange urgent removal to hospital.

TREATMENT

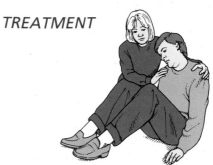

1 If the casualty is conscious, gently support and place him in a half-sitting position with his head and shoulders supported and his knees bent.

DO NOT let him move unnecessarily as this will put extra strain on his heart.

2 Loosen any constricting clothing around his neck, chest and waist.

3 Check breathing rate (see p.12), pulse (see p.85) and level of responsiveness (see p.95) at 10-minute intervals.

4 If he becomes unconscious, open his airway and check breathing. Complete the ABC of Resuscitation if required and place him in the Recovery Position (see pp.14–25).

5 Arrange urgent medical aid or removal to hospital. Transport as a stretcher case, maintaining the treatment position.

CARDIAC ARREST

This is a very serious condition in which the heart suddenly stops beating altogether. It can be the result of an extensive coronary obstruction.

SYMPTOMS & SIGNS

- Casualty will become unconscious.
- Breathing will be absent.
- Skin will be ashen.
- No pulse will be felt after two inflations of artificial ventilation.

AIM

Begin resuscitation without delay. Arrange urgent removal to hospital, making it clear that a heart attack is suspected.

TREATMENT

1 Begin resuscitation immediately (see pp.14–25).

2 Remove to hospital urgently. If necessary, continue resuscitation on the way.

STROKE

This term is used to describe a condition in which the blood supply to part of the brain is suddenly and critically impaired by a blood clot (cerebral thrombosis) or when a ruptured artery leaks blood into the brain (cerebral haemorrhage). The latter is more likely in people who have high blood pressure. In either case, the affected brain cells cease to function altogether.

Each area of the brain controls a different system or part of the body, and any deficiency resulting from a stroke depends on how much, and which part, of the brain is affected. Major strokes are often fatal, but many people make successful recoveries from minor strokes. Strokes are more common in people over 55, in those who are known to suffer from blackouts or circulatory disorders or in those who have had previous strokes. The symptoms and signs may be confused with drunkenness.

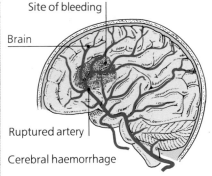

Site of bleeding

Brain

Ruptured artery

Cerebral haemorrhage

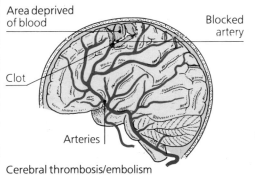

Area deprived of blood

Blocked artery

Clot

Arteries

Cerebral thrombosis/embolism

SYMPTOMS & SIGNS
- Possible sudden severe headache or giddiness.
- A strong pulse.
- Casualty may be disorientated, confused, anxious or weeping.
- Progressive loss of consciousness.

Depending on the extent of the stroke, one or more of the following physical defects may be also apparent:
- Paralysis of mouth – the corner of the mouth may droop, saliva may dribble from it, and speech may be slurred.
- Weakness and decreased sensation in one or both limbs and on one side of the body.
- Flushed face with hot, dry skin.
- Pupils may be unequal.
- Loss of bladder and bowel control.

AIM
Minimize the effects of damage to the brain and arrange urgent removal to hospital.

TREATMENT
1 If the casualty is conscious, lay him down with head and shoulders slightly raised and supported. Position his head on the side to allow saliva to drain from the mouth.

2 Loosen any constricting clothing around neck, chest and waist to assist circulation and breathing.

DO NOT give the casualty anything by mouth.

3 If the casualty becomes unconscious, open his airway and check breathing. Complete the ABC of Resuscitation if required and place him in the Recovery Postion (see pp.14–25).

4 Arrange urgent removal to hospital. Transport as a stretcher case, maintaining the treatment position.

UNCONSCIOUSNESS

The movements and functions of the body and the levels of responsiveness are governed by the nervous system.

Partial consciousness or unconsciousness in a casualty indicates that there is an interruption of the normal activity of the brain, which can be dangerous to the casualty. There are many causes of unconsciousness, the most common of which are: head injury, fainting, heart attack, stroke, asphyxia, epilepsy, shock, poisoning, infantile convulsions and diabetes.

The nervous system

This system comprises the brain, spinal cord and nerves.

The brain is an extremely delicate structure made up of a mass of nerve cells. It is here that sensations are analyzed and orders are given to the muscles. The brain is encased in the skull and suspended in clear (cerebro-spinal) fluid, which acts as a partial shock absorber. Nonetheless, since it is free to move within the skull, the brain is sensitive to violent movement or pressure.

The spinal cord is a mass of nerve fibres extending from the brain through an opening in the base of the skull. The cord runs through the spinal column (see p.124).

The peripheral nerves emerge in pairs, each containing motor and sensory nerves, from the brain and spinal cord. Sensory nerves transport impressions received by the senses (sight, hearing, touch, etc.) to the brain and motor nerves then transport the "orders" given by the brain to the voluntary muscles (see p.129). When a nerve is cut, there is a loss of feeling, power and movement in that part of the body controlled by the damaged nerve.

If the body is subjected to a stimulus, e.g., when touching a hot object, a so-called "reflex action" will attempt to remove the affected part of the body from the stimulus quickly by by-passing the normal pathway to and from the brain.

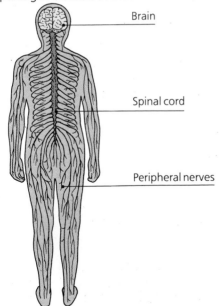

Brain

Spinal cord

Peripheral nerves

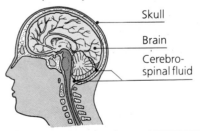

Skull

Brain

Cerebro-spinal fluid

The autonomic system
This is the network of nerves which controls the involuntary muscles – the muscles which regulate the vital functions of the body such as circulation, respiration and digestion. This system is not controlled by the will, and acts continuously whether a person is awake or asleep.

CHECKING FOR UNCONSCIOUSNESS

A conscious person is aware of himself and his surroundings whereas someone who is unconscious may not be completely aware of his surroundings. Unconsciousness is the result of an interruption of the normal activity of the brain. If the casualty does not respond normally to questions or conversation (e.g., What happened? What is your name? What is your address?) or does so only vaguely or inappropriately, he or she is in a state of altered consciousness and must be observed and treated accordingly.

The seriousness of the condition can be gauged by testing the casualty's response to stimuli such as sound, touch or pain. If he or she responds well to stimuli, the unconsciousness is only light, but the casualty is in a potentially dangerous state. If response is poor or absent, the unconsciousness is deeper and the risk correspondingly greater (see opposite).

Causes

There are many causes of unconsciousness and it can occur as a result of:
- Head injury, giving rise to concussion or compression.
- Disturbance of the blood supply to the brain as in fainting, heart attack, shock or stroke.
- Disturbance of the chemical content of the blood, e.g., lack of oxygen as in asphyxia; abnormal blood sugar as in diabetes; or presence of poison as in drug taking.
- Disturbance of the electrical activity of the brain, giving rise to fits.

NOTE

Diagnosing the cause of unconsciousness may be difficult or impossible for the First Aider, but this *must not* deter or delay treatment of the unconscious state.

GENERAL TREATMENT

The most important function of the First Aider is to ensure that the casualty's air passages remain open and clear, and that he or she is breathing adequately. It is also important to observe and take note of any alteration in the state of unconsciousness – either improving or deteriorating.

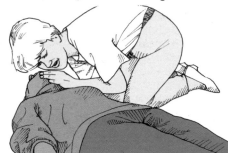

1 Open the casualty's air passages with jaw lift and head tilt (see p. 14). Remove any obvious obstruction. Loosen tight clothing. Check the breathing (see p. 15). If required, continue the ABC of Resuscitation (see pp. 14-25).

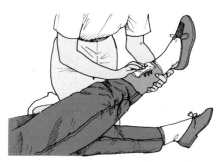

2 Examine the casualty quickly for serious injury. Control any severe bleeding or support any suspected fractures.

3 Assess level of responsiveness (see opposite), check breathing rate (see p. 12) and pulse (see p. 85).

4 Complete treatment of serious wounds and fractures.

5 Examine the casualty for less serious injuries or possible cause of unconsciousness. The presence of needle marks, warning bracelets, lockets or cards (see p.38) may be significant.

6 Place the casualty in the Recovery Position (see p.24). (A blanket may be placed under her whilst turning her.)

NOTE
If spinal injury is suspected, the casualty's airway still has priority. Extra care must be taken in turning such a casualty to maintain the normal neutral position of the spine. The normal recovery position cannot be used. *The Spinal Injury Recovery Position (see p.96) must be adopted for all unconscious casualties with suspected spinal injury.*

7 Cover the casualty with a blanket.

8 Remove her to hospital urgently, maintaining the Recovery Position.

9 If removal to hospital will be delayed, continue to check the level of responsiveness, breathing and pulse rate at least every 10 minutes. A written report of each assessment, including the time it was made, should be given to the doctor or ambulance attendant – this could govern the treatment eventually given (see *V.A.S. Observation Chart*, p.215).

DO NOT attempt to give an unconscious casualty anything by mouth.
DO NOT leave the casualty unattended.

IF the casualty recovers consciousness, reassure and observe her. Advise her to see a doctor.

ASSESSMENT OF LEVEL OF RESPONSIVENESS

This is adapted from the Glasgow Coma Scale which is internationally recognized and is in use in most hospitals throughout the United Kingdom. It is based upon eye opening, verbal and motor responses, and is a practical means of monitoring changes in the level of consciousness.

What follows is a simplified version of this method of assessment for First Aiders. See *V.A.S. Observation Chart*, p.215.

Note the time and response to the following:

EYES	MOVEMENT	SPEECH
■ Are they open?	■ Does the casualty move on command?	■ Is response to question and conversation normal?
■ Do they open on command?	■ Does the casualty move in response to painful stimuli?	■ Is the casualty confused?
■ Do they open in response to pain, e.g., pinching skin on back of hand?	■ Does the casualty make no response?	■ Does the casualty use inappropriate words?
■ Do they remain closed?		■ Does the casualty make incomprehensible sounds?
		■ Does the casualty make no response?

SUSPECTED FRACTURE OF THE SPINE

Certain accidents are especially associated with spinal injuries. These include falling from a height, weights falling on the spine, road traffic accidents, rugby, gymnastics, trampoline, equestrian and diving accidents.

When treating an unconscious casualty, you should be aware of the possibility that he or she may have fractured the spine. If a witness's description suggests that the casualty suffered a violent forward bending, backward bending or twisting injury of the spine, or if the distribution of the injuries suggests the possibility of a fractured spine, (e.g., wounds of the forehead often accompany injury to the cervical spine), you must assume that the force rendering the casualty unconscious has injured the spine until proved otherwise by X-ray. To protect the airway, put the casualty in the Spinal Injury Recovery Position as early as possible.

SPINAL INJURY RECOVERY POSITION

When adopting this position, take extra care to ensure that the casualty's spinal cord is not further injured. Ideally, six people are needed to move the casualty. All movements should be made at the command of the person holding the casualty's head.

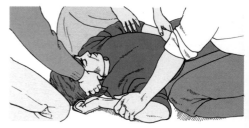

3 The helpers should straighten the casualty's legs, and place his arm on the side of the three helpers alongside his head, and the other arm to his side.

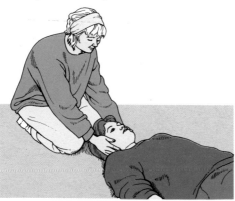

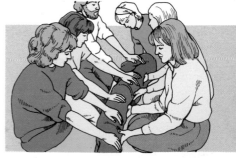

1 If possible, carefully place the casualty's head and neck in the normal neutral position (nose, navel and toes in line), and gently but firmly maintain this position by placing your hands over his ears.

2 Ask three helpers to kneel along one side of his trunk, and two on the other side.

4 The three helpers should place their arms over the casualty and log roll him to them on to his side as the other two gently lift him.

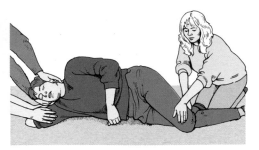

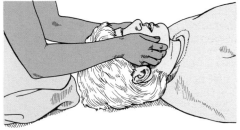

IF NO HELPERS ARE AVAILABLE

1 If his breathing is not difficult and his airway is clear, support the casualty in the position he was found until help arrives.

5 One helper should bend the casualty's lowermost arm under his head to further support his head and neck. Another helper should stabilize his trunk by bending his uppermost leg with his foot resting on the calf of his lowermost leg.

6 Continue to support his head and neck in the normal neutral position with your hands until skilled help arrives.

7 Without disturbing the head, apply a neck collar (see p.127) for added stability, when possible.

NOTE
During transport to hospital, continue to support the head and neck in the normal neutral position. Your hands are the most important means of support.

2 If his breathing becomes difficult, with minimal movement attempt to open the airway and keep it open by gently lifting the lower jaw forwards and up (jaw lift), keeping his head and neck in the normal neutral position.

3 If breathing is still difficult, tilt the head back *very slightly* (head tilt).

IF this does not restore adequate breathing or he vomits, place the casualty at once in the Spinal Injury Recovery Position to protect his airway. Continue to support his head and neck with your hands, and avoid twisting his spine (see pp.125–128). Apply a neck collar for additional stability when possible.

UNCONSCIOUS CASUALTY IN A CRASHED VEHICLE

If a casualty is found in a crashed vehicle, assume that he or she has a fracture of the spine (most probably the cervical spine) until proved otherwise.

DO NOT attempt to move the casualty unless it is absolutely necessary, e.g., he or she is in further danger, or requires external chest compression.

1 With your hands support his head and neck in the normal neutral position and maintain an open airway.

2 Carefully and gently apply a neck collar (see p.127) to give additional support to his head and neck.

IF the casualty has to be moved, four people are needed – one responsible for the head and neck, one for the shoulders and chest, one for the hips and abdomen, and one for the legs. The person supporting the head and neck directs movement.

HEAD INJURIES

These can result in damage to, or disturbance of, the brain. If this occurs, then the casualty's consciousness may be clouded or lost, concussion or compression may result and other associated injuries or conditions may be masked. A thorough examination of the casualty is, therefore, essential (see pp.33–36).

Direct blows to the head, heavy enough to cause scalp wounds or bruising, may be accompanied by skull fractures. This type of injury must receive urgent medical attention (see *Skull Fracture*, p.100, and *Scalp Wound*, p.69). A skull fracture may be present with little evidence of external damage.

These injuries commonly result from falls, particularly with intoxicated people; road accidents; sporting activities; or work in high-risk occupations such as construction work or mining.

CONCUSSION

This is a condition of widespread but temporary disturbance of the brain, sometimes described as "brain-shaking". It can result from a blow to the head, a fall from a height or a blow on the jaw.

Concussion can also occur *without* apparent unconsciousness. In some cases unconsciousness may have been so brief that the casualty may be unaware of, or have forgotten, the initial incident. *It is important to observe the casualty closely after any incident involving injury to the head.* If symptoms persist or the casualty's condition deteriorates, refer to a doctor without delay.

SYMPTOMS & SIGNS
■ Brief or partial loss of consciousness.
While the casualty is unconscious
■ Breathing may be shallow.
■ Face may be pale.
■ Skin may be cold and clammy.
■ Pulse may be rapid and weak.
During recovery
■ Casualty may feel nauseated or vomit.
On recovering consciousness
■ Casualty may not remember any events just before or after the incident. Ask the date, time, location. If he or she is unable to answer correctly, suspect concussion.

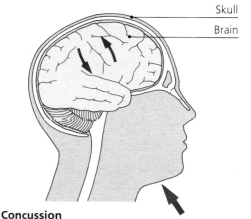

Skull

Brain

Concussion
When the head receives a blow the brain may "shake" within the skull.

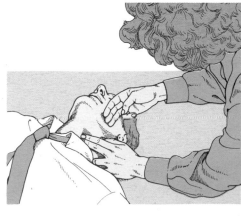

AIM
Treat any unconsciousness and obvious wounds and seek medical aid.

TREATMENT

1 In cases with apparent recovery, place the casualty in the care of a responsible person and advise him to consult a doctor.

2 Carry out the general treatment for the unconscious casualty where it is relevant.

3 Check breathing rate (see p.12), pulse rate (see p.85) and level of responsiveness (see p.95); watch carefully for signs of compression (see below) even after the casualty has apparently recovered.

4 Even if the casualty was unconscious for only a short time or you are unsure of his condition, arrange removal to hospital.

5 If unconsciousness persists or deepens, suspect compression and treat as below.

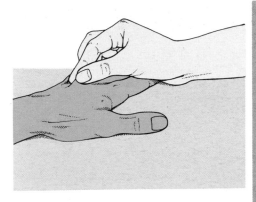

A test for responsiveness
Pinch the skin on the back of the casualty's hand to see if he responds to pain (see p.95).

COMPRESSION

This is a very serious condition in which pressure is exerted on the brain by blood accumulating within the skull or, occasionally, by pressure from bone in a depressed fracture (see p.100), or by swelling of the damaged brain. Compression can thus follow concussion and it may develop some hours or days after the casualty has apparently recovered.

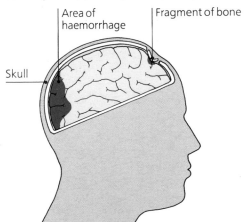

Area of haemorrhage Fragment of bone

Skull

Causes of compression
A blow may produce a depressed fracture and/or a build-up of blood in the skull. Either puts pressure on the brain.

SYMPTOMS & SIGNS
As compression develops, the casualty's level of responsiveness deteriorates.
■ Breathing may become noisy.
■ Pulse may be full and strong but slow.
■ Pupils may be of different sizes.
■ There may be weakness or paralysis of one side of the body.
■ Body temperature may rise, the face may become flushed but remain dry.

AIM
Arrange urgent removal to hospital.

TREATMENT

1 Carry out the general treatment for the unconscious casualty.

2 Treat shock from associated injuries (see p.86).

3 Arrange urgent removal to hospital, maintaining the Recovery Position.

NOTE
It is important that a good airway be maintained to ensure an adequate oxygen supply to the compressed brain. This reduces developing compression.

SKULL FRACTURES

The skull comprises a vault and a base. It provides a protective case for the brain, which is cushioned by a clear, watery fluid (cerebro-spinal fluid).

Fractures of the skull are important in so far as they indicate injury to the underlying brain, causing concussion or bruising (contusion), or because of bleeding which may occur beneath the fractured skull, causing pressure on the brain (compression). Occasionally a depressed fragment of skull, e.g., from a direct blow, may press on the brain. A fracture of the base of the skull is usually caused by indirect force as may occur in motor cycle accidents, when the helmeted head strikes an obstacle or the road, or as a result of a fall from a height.

SYMPTOMS & SIGNS

Fractures of the skull are most often diagnosed only by X-ray. However, the following may be present:
- Symptoms and signs of concussion and possibly compression.
- A soft boggy area or depression of the scalp revealed by gentle examination.
- With a fracture of the base, cerebro-spinal fluid and/or blood may leak from the casualty's nose or ear; there may be blood staining of the white of the eye; or the pupils may be different sizes.

AIM

Arrange urgent removal to hospital, making sure that an adequate airway is maintained.

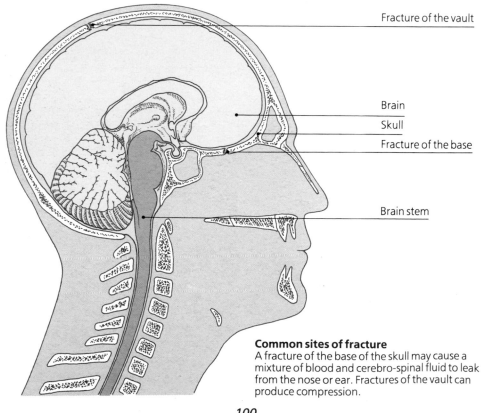

Fracture of the vault

Brain

Skull

Fracture of the base

Brain stem

Common sites of fracture
A fracture of the base of the skull may cause a mixture of blood and cerebro-spinal fluid to leak from the nose or ear. Fractures of the vault can produce compression.

TREATMENT

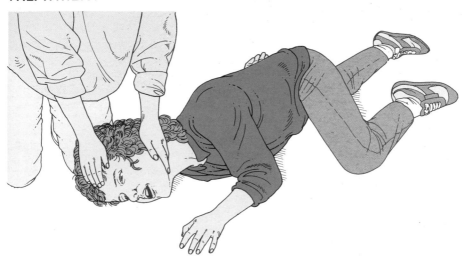

1 Turn the casualty carefully and gently into the Recovery Position (see p.24).

2 If there is discharge from one ear, turn her so that the affected ear is lower.

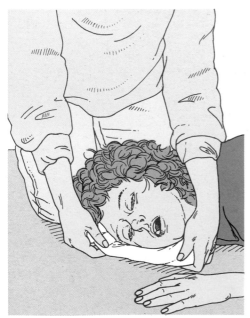

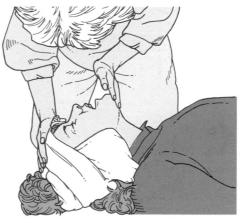

4 If she becomes unconscious, open her airway and check breathing. Complete the ABC of Resuscitation if necessary (see pp.14–25).

5 Check her breathing rate (see p.12), pulse (see p.85) and level of responsiveness (see p.95) at 10-minute intervals. Watch carefully for signs of compression (see p.99).

6 Arrange urgent removal to hospital.

3 Cover, but do *not* plug, the ear with a soft clean pad and bandage lightly.

IF a fracture of the spine is suspected, see p.125.

EPILEPSY

This is a condition which results from a tendency towards brief disruptions in the normal electrical activity of the brain. Epileptic fits may vary from momentary inattention without loss of consciousness (minor epilepsy) to muscular spasm and convulsions (major epilepsy).

MINOR EPILEPSY

This type of fit may start in childhood and may persist into adulthood. It can pass unnoticed because the casualty often appears only to be daydreaming.

SYMPTOMS & SIGNS
■ Casualty may appear to be in a daydream and be staring ahead blankly.
■ Casualty might start behaving strangely; these "automatisms" include chewing or smacking lips, saying odd things, or fiddling with clothing.
■ Casualty may have lost memory.

AIM
Protect the casualty while consciousness is impaired.

TREATMENT
1 Protect the casualty from any dangers such as busy roads. Keep other people away from him. Talk to him quietly.

2 Stay with him until you are certain that he has recovered and can get home.

NOTE
It is not unusual for a major fit to follow a minor one.

3 Advise the casualty to see a doctor.

MAJOR EPILEPSY

Most major epileptic attacks come on unexpectedly. However, sometimes a person experiences an *aura* which serves as a warning that something more severe is about to happen. The aura may differ from one person to another, e.g., a strange feeling in the body or a particular smell or taste. During an aura a person's normal mood may be altered, although this will not last long.

SYMPTOMS & SIGNS
During the fit
■ Casualty suddenly loses consciousness and falls to the ground, sometimes letting out a strange cry.
■ The casualty becomes rigid for a few seconds and breathing may cease. Mouth and lips will turn blue (cyanosis) and there will be congestion about the face and neck.

■ The muscles then relax and begin convulsive or jerking movements. These convulsions may be quite vigorous.
■ During this stage the breathing may be difficult or noisy through the clenched jaw; froth may appear around the mouth – it may be bloodstained if lips or tongue have been bitten; and there may be loss of control of the bladder and occasionally the bowel.
■ Finally, the muscles will relax although the casualty will remain unconscious for a few minutes or more.
After the fit is over
Usually no more than five minutes later, breathing will return to normal and the casualty will regain consciousness but may be dazed and confused and act strangely. This can last from several minutes to an hour and the person may want to rest quietly.

AIM

Protect the casualty from injury during the fit and provide care once he or she has regained consciousness.

TREATMENT

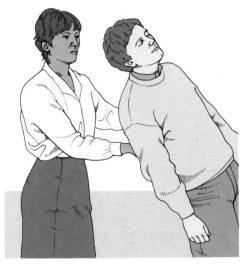

1 If the casualty is falling, try to support him or ease his fall and lay him down gently, in a safe place if possible.

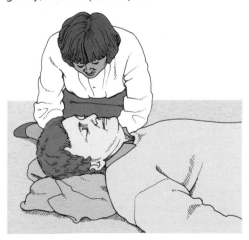

2 Clear a space around him and, unless you want someone to help, ask all bystanders to leave. If possible, carefully loosen clothing around his neck and place something soft under his head.

DO NOT move or lift the casualty unless in danger.

DO NOT forcibly restrain him.

DO NOT put anything in his mouth or try to open it.

DO NOT try to wake the casualty.

3 When the convulsions cease, place the casualty in the Recovery Position to aid his breathing (see p.24).

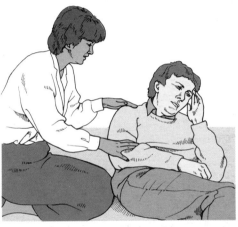

4 When the attack is over stay with the casualty until you are certain recovery is complete.

DO NOT give the casualty anything to drink until you are sure of full alertness.

5 Even if he makes a full, quick recovery, advise him to inform his doctor about the latest attack.

DO NOT send for an ambulance unless the casualty has several fits, has been injured during the fit or takes longer than 15 minutes to regain consciousness. If he has an epilepsy card, it may tell you how long he normally takes to wake up.

CONVULSIONS IN INFANTS AND CHILDREN

In children under the age of five, a raised temperature caused by the onset of an infectious disease or a throat or ear infection can cause convulsions. Despite their alarming nature, they are rarely dangerous but the signs may persist while the child's temperature remains abnormally high.

SYMPTOMS & SIGNS
- Child has high fever and may be "flushed" and sweating.
- Twitching of muscles of face and limbs.
- Occasional squinting or upturned eyes.
- There may be stiffness or rigidity, with the head back and spine arched.
- Child may be holding his or her breath.
- Congestion of the face and neck.
- Froth may appear at the mouth.

AIM
Protect the child from injury and cool him or her to reduce the intensity of the fit. Seek medical aid and reassure the parents.

TREATMENT
1 Ensure a good supply of fresh air.

2 Loosen any constricting clothing around the child's neck and chest.

3 Clear a space around the child if the convulsions are severe.

4 Carry out the general treatment for the unconscious casualty.

5 Cool the child: first remove any covering bedclothes and/or clothes, then sponge him or her with tepid water, starting from the head and working down.

DO NOT allow the child to become too chilled.

6 Reassure the child's parents and advise them to seek medical aid.

HYSTERIA

This is usually caused by an over-reaction to an emotional upset or nervous stress and is likely to be heightened by the presence of any onlookers.

SYMPTOMS & SIGNS
- Temporary loss of behavioural control with dramatic shouting, screaming, crying, and/or wild beating of limbs. Casualty may be rolling around on the ground and/or tearing at hair and clothes.
- Hysterical over-breathing (hyper-ventilation) may follow.
- Casualty may be unwilling to move or be making strange movements.

AIM
Isolate the casualty from any onlookers and, gently but firmly, help him or her to calm down enough to regain control.

TREATMENT
1 Reassure the casualty, refrain from showing him or her any sympathy and, gently, but firmly, escort to a quiet place.

DO NOT physically restrain or slap the casualty; this may make him or her behave more violently.

2 Stay with the casualty and keep under observation until fully recovered.

3 Advise the casualty to see a doctor.

EMERGENCIES IN DIABETES

Diabetes (diabetes mellitus) is a condition which arises when there is a disturbance in the way the body regulates the sugar concentrations in the blood. This can result in two conditions: too much sugar in the blood (hyperglycaemia) or too little sugar in the blood (hypoglycaemia). If prolonged, both conditions can result in unconsciousness and eventually, the death of the casualty. However, hyperglycaemia normally develops very gradually so it is rare for a First Aider to find a casualty in this condition.

Diabetics need to control their blood sugar levels carefully by balancing the amount of sugar in their diets with insulin injections or tablets. Most diabetics, including children, give their own treatments two or three times a day, and eat an appropriate amount of the correct types of food. As a result many carry hypodermic needles, insulin bottles or other medication on them all the time. Most diabetics also carry a card or wear a bracelet (see p.38) indicating that they have diabetes.

LOW BLOOD SUGAR (HYPOGLYCAEMIA)

If a diabetic has taken too much insulin by mistake, has eaten too little food or missed a meal, or if exercise has burned up the sugar, the concentration of sugar in the blood falls. Low blood sugar will affect the brain and, if prolonged or very low, it will result in unconsciousness and the possible death of the casualty.

SYMPTOMS & SIGNS

- A diabetic may feel faint, dizzy and light-headed and may be aware that his or her sugar level is low.
- Casualty may be confused and disorientated and may appear to be drunk and possibly aggressive.
- Skin becomes pale, with profuse sweating.
- Pulse becomes rapid.
- Breathing becomes shallow and breath will be odourless.
- Limbs may begin to tremble.

- Casualty's level of responsiveness may deteriorate rapidly.

NOTE
The longer a diabetic has been on insulin the less evident the early warning symptoms may become so it may be difficult for you to diagnose the casualty's condition.

AIM
Restore the sugar/insulin balance as soon as possible. If the casualty is unconscious, arrange urgent removal to hospital.

TREATMENT

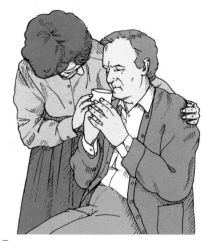

IF the casualty is conscious and capable of swallowing, immediately give sugar lumps, a sugary drink, chocolate or other sweet food in order to raise the level of sugar in the blood. If the condition improves within a few minutes, give more sweetened food or drink. Instruct the casualty to seek medical advice.

IF the casualty is unconscious, carry out the general treatment for the unconscious casualty. Seek medical aid and arrange urgent removal to hospital.

FRACTURES

A fracture is a broken or cracked bone. Bones behave like the branches of a tree when struck, twisted or strained. Generally, considerable force is required to break a bone, but old bones – like old trees – break more easily. Conversely, young bones are supple and may split, bend or crack under stress just like a young sapling.

All fractures should be handled carefully as undue movement may cause further damage to surrounding blood vessels or organs.

Fractures may be caused by either direct or indirect force.

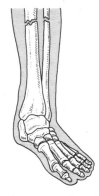

Direct force
A bone may fracture at a point where severe force is applied. For example, if someone is struck by a moving vehicle, their leg bones may be broken by the direct impact of a car bumper, or a blow from a footballer's boot could cause a fracture.

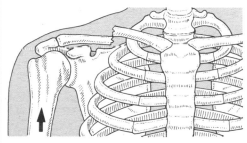

Indirect force
A bone may also fracture some distance from the point of impact. For example, after a fall on an outstretched hand, the force may be transmitted along the whole length of the upper limb so that the collar-bone breaks.

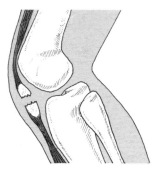

Another type of indirect fracture occurs when a muscle pulls violently on an attached bone causing it to fracture. For example, when a footballer kicks the ground instead of the ball, the sudden contraction of the powerful thigh muscle may break the attached kneecap.

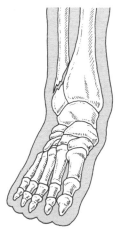

A third form of indirect fracture occurs when a twisting or wrenching force causes a rotating strain to be transmitted to an attached bone and breaks it. For example, if the foot is twisted when someone trips, the strain may fracture the bones of the leg.

The skeleton

The body is built on a framework of bones called the skeleton. This skeleton supports the muscles, blood vessels and nerves of the body and gives protection to certain organs, e.g., the skull protects the brain, while the ribcage and breastbone protect the heart, lungs and other vital organs. Movement of the body is made possible by bones and their attached muscles.

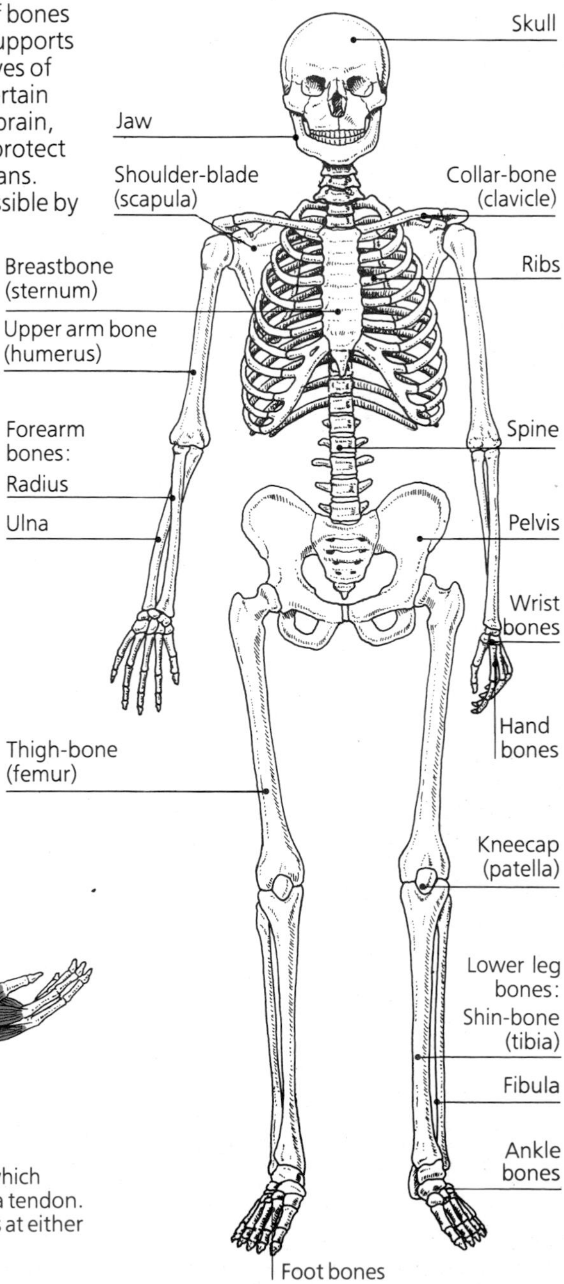

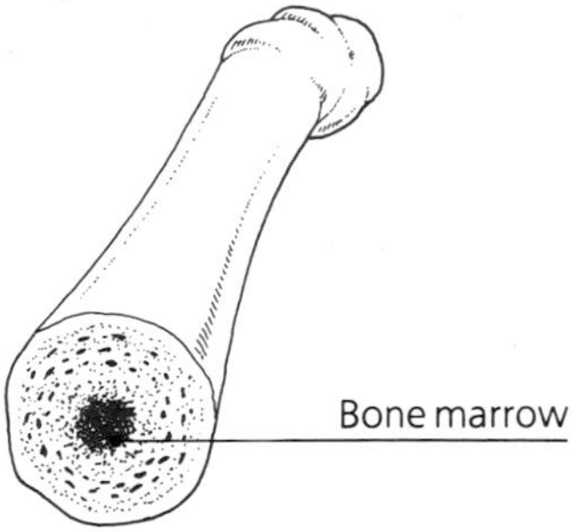

Bone marrow

Cross-section of a bone
A bone consists of a hardened outer layer and softer centre, called marrow, through which blood vessels travel and where blood cells are formed.

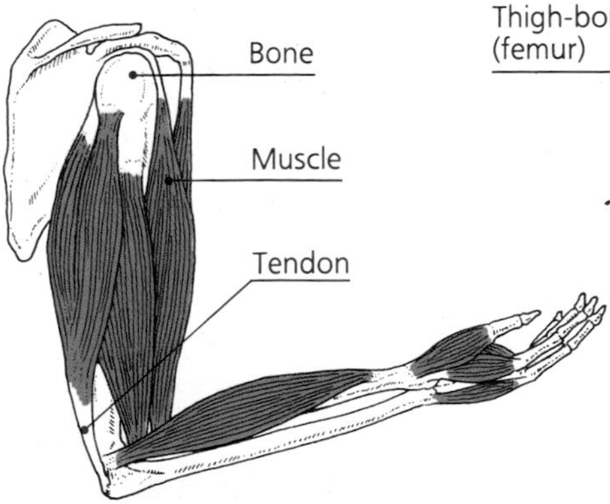

Bone

Muscle

Tendon

How muscles are attached
Most muscles consist of a fleshy belly which narrows down to a fibrous cord called a tendon. This fibrous tissue attaches the muscles at either end to bones.

Skull

Jaw

Shoulder-blade (scapula)

Collar-bone (clavicle)

Breastbone (sternum)

Ribs

Upper arm bone (humerus)

Forearm bones:

Radius

Ulna

Spine

Pelvis

Wrist bones

Hand bones

Thigh-bone (femur)

Kneecap (patella)

Lower leg bones:
Shin-bone (tibia)

Fibula

Ankle bones

Foot bones

TYPES OF FRACTURE

There are two main types of fracture, closed or open.

Closed fracture
With this type of fracture the skin surface which envelops the fractured bone is not broken. However, considerable damage may be done to surrounding muscles and blood vessels, causing the affected part to swell due to internal bleeding.

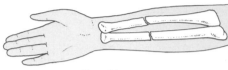

Closed fracture

Open fracture
In open fractures the overlying skin is broken so that the fractured bone, or bones, are in direct communication with the surface and surrounding environment. Bleeding will be evident and there is great danger of infection from contamination entering the site of the fracture.

Open fractures may occur from within, where fragments break outwards through the skin, or from without, e.g., through a missile wound or when someone is struck by a car or machinery.

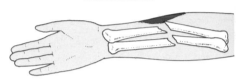

Open fracture

NOTE
Both closed and open fractures may be *complicated* by injury to blood vessels, nerves or adjacent organs by fractured bone ends or fragments.

GENERAL SYMPTOMS & SIGNS
■ The snap of the bone may have been felt or heard by the casualty.
■ Pain at or near the site of injury increased by movement.
■ Casualty may find it difficult or impossible to move the part normally.
■ Tenderness at the site of the fracture when gentle pressure is applied over the affected area. Do not touch an open fracture site.
■ Swelling and, later, bruising of the injured part. This may not be evident at first but will develop as blood leaks into the tissues; it may mask the true nature of the injury.
■ Deformity at the site of the fracture. This may be irregularity of the bone; shortening, angulation or rotation of the limb (e.g., the limb has twisted further than is normally possible – a turned out foot is common with a fractured thigh-bone), or depression of a flat bone may occur.

■ Coarse bony grating (crepitus) may be heard or felt upon examination – this should *never* be sought deliberately.
■ Symptoms and signs of shock (see p.86). The degree of shock will be particularly noticeable in those with a fractured thigh-bone or pelvis.

NOTE
Not all the symptoms and signs will be present in every fracture. As many as possible should be noted by simple observation without moving any part unnecessarily. Compare the shape of the injured and uninjured limbs whenever possible. If you are in any doubt about the severity of an injury, treat as a fracture.

AIM

Prevent movement at the injured site and arrange removal to hospital.

GENERAL TREATMENT

Casualties with fractures should be treated initially at the site of the accident, warned to lie still, and not be moved until the affected part has been properly immobilized, unless life is in danger, e.g., from fire or falling buildings. If you do have to move the casualty, support the fractured limb (see below) and move as gently as possible to minimize pain and further injury. During treatment keep the casualty as comfortable as possible and protect from the cold.

> ### NOTE
> Difficulty in breathing, severe bleeding and unconsciousness must be dealt with *before* treating a fracture.

Specific fractures are considered later. However, the general principles of treatment of limb fractures are as follows:

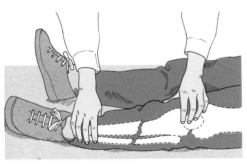

1 Steady and support the fractured limb by holding it with one hand above and one below the site of fracture. Keep holding the limb until it is effectively immobilized.

2 Immobilize the fractured bone by splintage. The most natural form of splintage is the casualty's own body. For upper limb fractures, apply padding and a sling, and bandage the arm to the trunk. For lower limb fractures, bandage the injured leg to the opposite leg. Bring the leg into line by moving the uninjured to the injured leg.

IF a fractured limb is bent or angled so severely as to prevent bringing it into line with its fellow, it is permissible to pull the limb straight. Do this by pulling very gently, applying traction in the long axis of the limb, i.e., along the line of the thigh-bone to shin-bone or upper arm to forearm bones. No harm will occur provided that you pull only in this straight line and use only gentle traction. Maintain traction until the limb is securely immobilized.

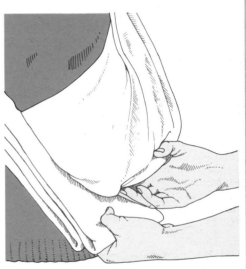

3 In splintage it is essential to place adequate padding between bony prominences, e.g., knees and ankles, and to fill hollows, e.g., between the arm and trunk.

4 When bandaging the limb, it is essential to immobilize the joints above and below the fractured site, e.g., the knee and ankle joints in the case of lower leg fractures.

5 Tie the bandages firmly enough to prevent movement, but not so tight as to interfere with the circulation of the limb. (Remember that swelling is likely to increase rapidly.) Check the circulation at intervals where possible (see p.175).

6 After immobilization, where possible, elevate the affected limb to minimize bleeding and swelling. Both legs may be elevated, e.g., by raising the foot of the stretcher, to minimize shock (see p.86).

OPEN FRACTURES

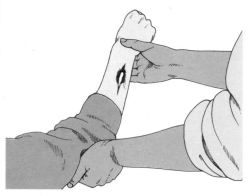

1 Steady, elevate and support the arm.

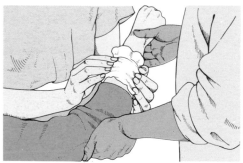

2 Place a piece of sterile gauze or suitable dressing over the wound and apply pressure to control bleeding.

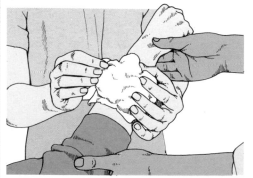

3 Place pads of cotton wool or similar material over and around the wound.

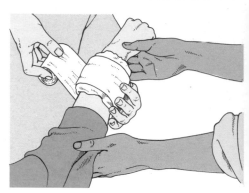

4 Secure dressing and padding with a firm bandage.

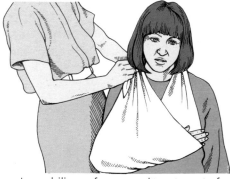

5 Immobilize as for general treatment of fracture and elevate the injured part, if possible.

6 Arrange removal to hospital, maintaining the treatment position. Transport as a stretcher case if necessary.

NOTE
If bone is protruding, build up the dressing and pads around the bone as for foreign bodies (see p.64).

Upper limbs

The *shoulder girdle* and *upper limbs* consist of the collar-bone (clavicle), the shoulder-blade (scapula, which is rarely broken) and the upper arm bone (humerus). The *collar-bone* is situated between the upper part of the breastbone and the shoulder, and forms a strut to hold the upper limbs away from the chest. The shoulder-blade forms joints with the collar-bone and the *upper arm bone*.

Each upper limb consists of the upper arm bone, the two bones in the forearm which allow for the turning action of the wrist, and the small bones at the wrist.

More bones form the framework of the palm of the hand and fingers and thumb.

COLLAR-BONE FRACTURES

These fractures are commonly caused by indirect force resulting from a fall on to an outstretched hand or the point of the shoulder. Collar-bone fractures due to direct force are rare.

SYMPTOMS & SIGNS
■ General symptoms and signs of fracture.
■ Pain and tenderness at the site of injury increased by movement.
■ Casualty is reluctant to move the limb on the injured side.
■ Casualty may support the arm on the injured side at the elbow and may incline the head towards the injured side to relax muscles and relieve pain.
■ Deformity may be seen or felt over the site of fracture.

AIM
Immobilize upper limb and remove casualty to hospital.

TREATMENT

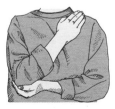

1 Sit the casualty down. Gently place the limb on her injured side across her chest with her fingertips almost resting on the opposite shoulder.

2 Support the limb in an elevation sling (see p.179).

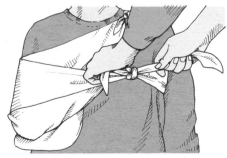

3 Place soft padding between her upper arm and chest on the affected side.

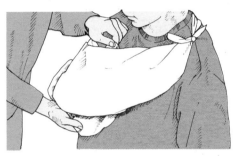

4 Secure the limb to her chest by applying a broad-fold bandage over the sling. Tie the knot in front on the uninjured side.

5 Arrange removal to hospital; transport as a sitting or walking case unless there are complications.

UPPER ARM & FOREARM FRACTURES

Fractures can occur anywhere along the length of the upper arm bone or the two forearm bones, and may involve the elbow. The bones most frequently broken, however, are those at the wrist.

Fractures involving the elbow joint are especially common in children. This fracture may cause extensive damage to the surrounding blood vessels and nerves.

SYMPTOMS & SIGNS
■ General symptoms and signs of fracture.
■ Pain at the site of fracture increased by movement.
■ Casualty is probably unable to use the arm.
■ Possible inability to bend or straighten the elbow of the injured arm.

AIM
Immobilize limb and remove to hospital.

UPPER ARM FRACTURE

1 Sit the casualty down. Gently support the forearm of the injured limb across his chest.

2 Support limb in an arm sling (see p.178).

3 Gently place soft padding between his upper arm and his chest.

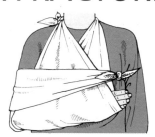

4 Secure the limb to his chest with a broad-fold bandage applied over the sling, close to the elbow (but preferably not over the site of the fracture). Tie the knot in front of the uninjured side. Check circulation (see p.175).

5 Arrange removal to hospital; transport in the sitting position.

FOREARM & WRIST FRACTURES

1 Sit the casualty down. Gently support the injured forearm and place across his chest.

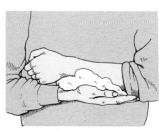

2 Gently cradle forearm in a fold of soft padding.

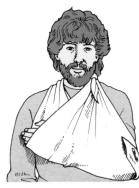

3 Support limb in an arm sling (see p.178).

4 Secure the limb to his chest with a broad-fold bandage applied over the sling, close to the elbow, preferably avoiding the site of fracture. Tie knot in front of the uninjured side. Check the casualty's circulation (see p.175).

5 Arrange removal to hospital; transport in the sitting position.

IF THE ELBOW CANNOT BE BENT OR THE CASUALTY IS LYING DOWN

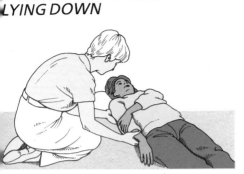

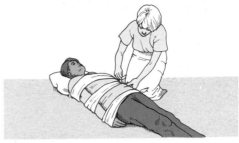

1 Lay the casualty down and support the injured limb by the side of her trunk. *Do not attempt to bend the elbow by force.*

2 Place adequate soft padding between the injured limb and her trunk, to ensure that application of bandages will not displace the broken bones.

3 Secure the injured limb to her body by three broad-fold bandages: around the wrist and hips; the upper arm and trunk; and the forearm and trunk at the elbow, preferably not over the fracture site. Tie knots on uninjured side. Check circulation (see p.175).

4 Arrange removal to hospital; transport as a stretcher case, maintaining the treatment position.

HAND & FINGER FRACTURES

Fractures of the hand are usually due to direct force. They can be caused by crushing and may involve severe bleeding.

SYMPTOMS & SIGNS
- General symptoms and signs of fracture.
- Casualty is unable to use fingers.
- Extensive swelling and bruising.

AIM
Immobilize the injured hand and arrange removal to hospital.

TREATMENT

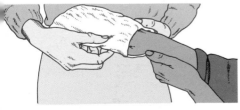

1 Protect the injured hand by placing it in a fold of soft padding.

2 Gently support the affected limb in an elevation sling (see p.179).

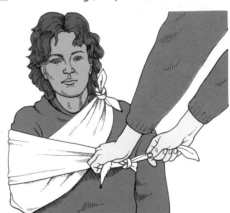

3 Secure the limb to the casualty's chest by applying a broad-fold bandage over the sling. Tie the knot in front of the uninjured side. Check circulation (see p.175).

4 Arrange removal to hospital; transport in the sitting position if possible.

Trunk

The *ribs* consist of 12 pairs of curved bones, most of which extend from the vertebrae round to the front of the body.

The *chest cavity* is bounded in front by the breastbone, behind by the spine, below by the diaphragm, then encircled by the ribs. It contains the heart and major blood vessels, the lungs and the gullet.

The *pelvis* is a basin-shaped structure of bone attached to the lower part of the spine. It supports and protects the contents of the lower abdominal cavity and contains sockets for the hip joints.

RIB & BREASTBONE FRACTURES

Rib fractures usually result from direct force, e.g., a blow to, or heavy fall on to, the chest, or from indirect force as a result of being crushed. If the fracture is complicated by a "sucking wound" of the chest (see p.76) or by "paradoxical breathing" due to a stove-in-chest (see p.54), asphyxia may result unless the injuries are treated immediately.

SYMPTOMS & SIGNS

- General symptoms and signs of fracture.
- Casualty feels a sharp pain at the site of the fracture, increased by anything more than shallow breathing or by coughing.
- Possible symptoms and signs of internal bleeding (see p.66) indicating damage to internal organs such as the lungs or liver.
- There may be an open wound of the chest wall over the fracture, causing a "sucking wound" of the chest.
- Possible paradoxical breathing if there are multiple fractures (see p.54).

AIM

Make the casualty as comfortable as possible and arrange removal to hospital.

TREATMENT

1 Support the limb on the injured side in an arm sling (see p.178).

2 Arrange removal to hospital; transport as a sitting or walking casualty unless there are complications.

FOR A COMPLICATED FRACTURE

1 Immediately treat any "sucking wound" (see p.76).

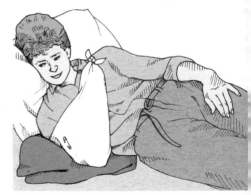

2 Lay the casualty down in a half-sitting position with his head and shoulders turned and his body inclined towards the injured side. Support him by placing a folded blanket lengthwise along his back.

3 Support the limb on the injured side in an elevation sling (see p.179).

4 If the casualty is unconscious or breathing becomes difficult and/or noisy, place him in the Recovery Position (see p.24) with his uninjured side uppermost.

5 Arrange removal to hospital; transport as a stretcher case, maintaining the treatment position.

114

PELVIC FRACTURES

These are usually caused by a direct crush injury or by indirect force such as might occur during vehicle collisions. For example, the impact of a car's fascia on a knee can force the head of the thigh-bone through the socket of the hip joint.

One or both sides of the pelvic girdle may be fractured and pelvic injuries can be complicated by injury to the bladder and urinary passages.

SYMPTOMS & SIGNS

- General symptoms and signs of fracture.
- Pain and tenderness in the region of the hips, groin or back, which is increased when the casualty moves.
- Casualty is unable to walk or even stand, although the legs appear sound.
- If the casualty passes water it may be bloodstained.
- Symptoms and signs of shock which may become severe (see p.86).

AIM

Make the casualty comfortable and arrange urgent removal to hospital.

TREATMENT

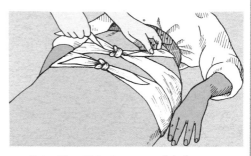

2 If the First Aider is responsible for transporting the casualty, gently apply two broad-fold bandages around her pelvis, the lower one first. Tie off in the centre. This measure is not always necessary and should not be carried out if it causes excessive pain.

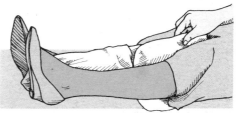

3 Place adequate soft padding between her knees and ankles.

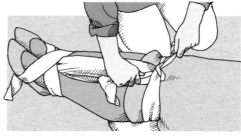

4 Apply a figure-of-eight bandage around her ankles and feet and a broad-fold bandage around her knees.

5 To minimize shock, cover her with a blanket.

6 Arrange removal to hospital; transport as a stretcher case, maintaining the treatment position.

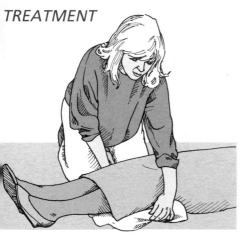

1 Place the casualty on her back with her legs straight or, if it is more comfortable for her, bend her knees slightly and place a rolled blanket underneath them.

Lower limbs

Each *lower limb* consists of: the thigh-bone (femur); the two bones of the lower leg, the shin-bone (tibia) and the fibula; and a number of smaller bones in the foot and ankle. The thigh-bone reaches from the hip to the knee and is the longest and strongest bone in the body. Its lower end forms part of the knee joint, and its head fits into the pelvis at the hip joint.

The *kneecap* (patella) is a small, flattish bone which lies in front of the knee joint. The two bones of the lower leg extend from the knee to the ankle; the long thin bone (fibula) lies on the outer side of the thicker shin-bone. A number of smaller bones make up the foot.

LOWER LEG FRACTURES

Either or both of the two bones of the lower leg, the shin-bone (tibia) and the fibula, may be broken. Fractures of the upper end of the shin-bone commonly occur when pedestrians are hit by car bumpers; they are known as "bumper" fractures. Shin-bone fractures are often open because only a thin layer of skin and tissue covers the bone.

The fibula is most commonly broken by "wrenching" of the ankle joint. However, because this is not a weight-bearing bone, a simple fracture is often mistaken for a severe sprain, especially if a crack fracture occurs a few inches above the ankle. As a result, the casualty may not seek medical advice until a few days after the injury.

SYMPTOMS & SIGNS
- General symptoms and signs of fracture.
- Swelling and bruising apparent.
- Angulation (bending) and rotation (twisting) may be seen.
- Deformity (irregularity) may be seen or felt along one or both bones.
- Possible "open" wound if shin-bone is fractured.
- Possible symptoms and signs of shock (see p.86).

AIM
Immobilize fracture and remove the casualty to hospital.

TREATMENT

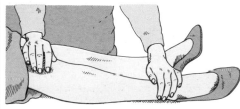

1 Lay the casualty down and carefully steady and support the limb by holding it at the joints above and below the site of the injury; get a bystander to do this if possible.

2 If necessary, gently expose the injured leg (cut clothing) and examine to identify the type of fracture (closed/open).

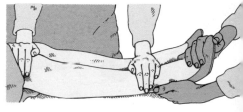

3 Holding her ankle and foot, apply gentle traction, carefully pulling in the long axis of the limb to bring the limb into its normal straight line.

IF arrival of the ambulance is imminent, maintain support of the limb until it arrives. Treat to minimize shock (see p.86).

4 Otherwise, whilst support of the limb is maintained at the ankle, using the natural hollows, gently place broad-fold bandages in position under the casualty's legs at the knees, and above and below the fracture and a narrow-fold bandage at the ankles.

NOTE
Gentle traction and support must be maintained continuously until immobilization is complete.

5 Gently bring her sound limb alongside the injured limb.

6 Place adequate soft padding between her legs to cover the bony prominences at the knees and ankles, and further padding to ensure that application of bandages does not displace broken bones.

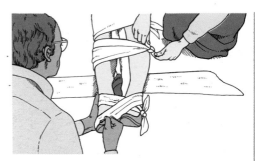

7 Tie the bandage at her ankles and feet in a figure-of-eight, and the other bandages around her knees, and above and below the fracture on the lower leg. Use gentle tension when applying bandages to ensure firmness. Avoid jerky movements. Tie the knots on the uninjured side.

IF the fracture is near the casualty's ankle, do not apply a bandage below the fracture; application of the figure-of-eight bandage should be modified to avoid bandaging over the fracture.

IF CASUALTY TO BE TRANSPORTED BY THE FIRST AIDER

1 Whilst the injured limb is in a straight line, supported by hand and traction (see opposite), using the natural hollows, gently place four broad-fold bandages in position under the legs at the thighs, knees, above and below the fracture on the lower leg, and a narrow-fold bandage at the ankles.

4 Place adequate soft padding between her legs to cover the bony prominences at her knees and ankles, and further padding in the hollows to ensure application of bandages does not displace broken bones.

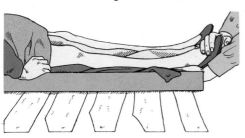

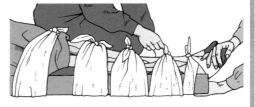

5 Secure the splint to the limbs by tying the bandage around the upper thighs. Tie the other bandages as in step 7 (above). Tie the knots on the uninjured side.

2 Place a splint with adequate padding along the outside of the fractured limb, extending from the casualty's upper thigh to her foot. Ensure further padding protects bony areas and that all hollows are filled.

3 Gently bring her sound limb alongside the injured limb.

NOTE
Gentle traction and support must be maintained continuously until immobilization is complete.

THIGH-BONE FRACTURES

A fracture can occur anywhere along the length of the thigh-bone (femur). It is the longest bone in the body and has a rich blood supply. All incidents where the thigh-bone is fractured should be regarded as serious because, in most cases, a large volume of blood is lost into the tissues and this may result in severe shock (see p.86).

This type of fracture often results from falls and road traffic accidents. In the aged a fracture may result from a minor fall; in most adults, however, considerable force is required to break the thigh-bone.

Fractures at the hip joint involving the neck or upper portion of the thigh-bone are often mistaken for a badly bruised hip. Any elderly person who complains of pain in the hip after a fall or other minor accident may have a fracture of the neck of the thigh-bone and should be removed to hospital.

SYMPTOMS & SIGNS
■ General symptoms and signs of fracture.
■ Visible deformity in lower limb: the limb may be shortened by contraction of muscles around fractured bone; the foot and kneecap may be turned outwards (rotation).
■ Symptoms and signs of shock (see p.86).

AIM
Immobilize fracture and remove casualty to hospital.

TREATMENT

1 Lay the casualty down and carefully steady and support his injured limb by holding it at the joints above and below the site of injury.

2 If necessary, gently expose the leg to identify type of fracture (closed/open).

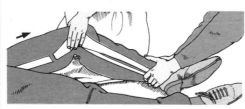

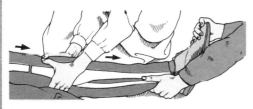

3 Apply gentle traction holding his knee. Whilst traction and support are continued at the knee, the assistant gently straightens the lower leg. Bring the injured leg into a straight line by continuing traction at the ankle, releasing traction at the knee.

IF arrival of the ambulance is imminent, maintain support until it arrives. Treat to minimize shock (see p.86).

4 Otherwise, whilst the injured limb is supported at the ankle, using the natural hollows, gently place broad-fold bandages in position under the casualty's legs at the knees and above and below the fracture, and a narrow-fold bandage at the ankles.

5 Gently bring his sound limb alongside the injured limb.

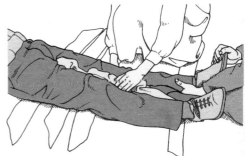

6 Place adequate soft padding between his legs to cover the bony prominences at the knees and ankles, and further padding to ensure that application of bandages does not displace broken bones.

7 Tie the bandage around his ankles and feet in a figure-of-eight, and the other bandages around his knees, then above and below the fracture on his thigh. Use gentle tension when applying bandages to ensure firmness. Avoid jerky movements. Tie the knots on the uninjured side.

NOTE
If the fracture is near to the knee or hip, it may be necessary to modify the positions of the bandages to avoid bandaging over it.

IF CASUALTY TO BE TRANSPORTED BY THE FIRST AIDER

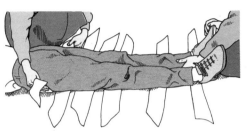

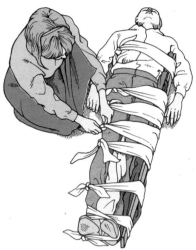

1 Whilst the injured limb is in a straight line, supported by hand and traction (as opposite), gently place four broad-fold bandages in position under the legs, above and below the fracture at the thighs, knees and lower legs, and a narrow-fold at the ankles. Using the natural hollow at his waist, place additional broad-fold bandages in position under the chest and pelvis.

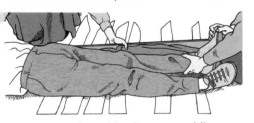

2 Place a splint with adequate padding along the outside of the fractured limb, extending from armpit to foot. Ensure further padding protects bony areas and that all hollows are filled.

3 Gently bring the sound limb alongside the injured limb.

4 Place adequate soft padding between the casualty's legs to cover bony prominences at his knees and ankles, and further padding in the hollows to ensure that application of bandages does not displace broken bones.

5 Secure the splint to his trunk by tying the bandages around his chest just below the armpits, and around his pelvis in line with his hip joints. Tie the other bandages in a figure-of-eight at ankles and feet, around knees, lower leg, and above and below the fractured site at the thigh. Use gentle tension when applying bandages to ensure firmness. Tie the knots on the uninjured side.

6 To minimize shock, treat as on p.86.

7 Arrange removal to hospital; transport as a stretcher case, maintaining the treatment position.

NOTE
In all cases of fracture of the lower limb, if possible raise the legs slightly (i.e., raise the lower end of the stretcher) to minimize swelling and shock.

KNEE JOINT INJURIES

The knee forms a hinge joint, which swings to and fro in one plane only. The lower end of the thigh-bone (femur) rests on the upper end of the shin-bone (tibia), the bones being connected by strong ligaments. Attached around the rim of the upper surface of the shin-bone are two thick, half-moon shaped cushions of cartilage. The knee joint is supported by strong muscles, and in front of the joint lies the kneecap (patella).

Any of these structures may be damaged by violent twists or strains. If the knee joint is forced sideways or backwards, ligaments may rupture. A rotational strain, whilst the weight of the body is on the same foot, often results in rupture and displacement of a cartilage. A direct blow or violent contraction of the attached muscle may dislocate or fracture the kneecap.

To the First Aider, the distinction between these differing injuries may be impossible, but this does not matter as the treatment is the same for them all.

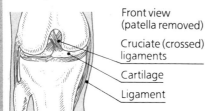

Front view (patella removed)

Cruciate (crossed) ligaments

Cartilage

Ligament

SYMPTOMS & SIGNS

■ Pain, which may be localized at first to the site of injury, but quickly becomes deep seated in the joint. All attempted movement of the joint is painful.
■ Possible local tenderness.
■ Rapid swelling of the joint due to internal bleeding.
■ Possible "locking" of the knee in a bent position.
■ Possible deformity with severe injuries.

AIM

Protect the knee in the most comfortable position, whilst transporting the casualty to hospital.

TREATMENT

DO NOT attempt to force the knee straight. There may be a displaced cartilage or internal bleeding from a ruptured ligament or fractured kneecap, which makes the knee joint tense and impossible to straighten.

1 If she is standing, do not allow the casualty to walk. Help her to lie down on her back and support her leg in the most comfortable position.

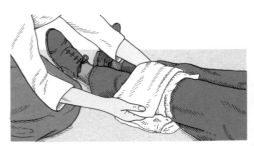

2 Bandaging is not essential but for comfort and protection, place soft padding around the joint. Bandage carefully, allowing for swelling.

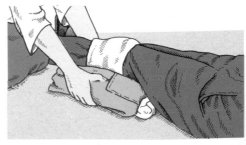

3 Support the knee by placing a small pillow, folded blanket or coat underneath. Give nothing by mouth.

4 Carry the casualty by stretcher to ambulance. Transport to hospital, maintaining the treatment position.

FOOT FRACTURES

Fractures of the foot often result from direct injuries, such as being run over or hit or crushed by heavy objects. However, injury can result from twisting falls or jumps.

SYMPTOMS & SIGNS
■ General symptoms and signs of fracture.
■ Pain in foot increased by movement.
■ Loss of movement of foot; casualty unable to walk properly on foot.

■ Tenderness at fracture site.
■ Swelling and bruising may be present at site of injury.
■ Deformity, such as irregularity of the bony arch may be present.

AIM
Minimize swelling in the injured foot and arrange removal to hospital.

TREATMENT
1 Lay the casualty down.

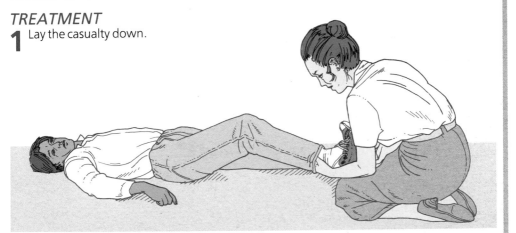

2 Support the foot and gently remove footwear.

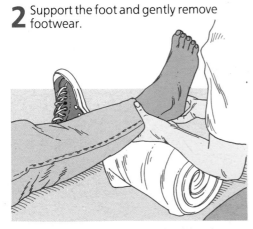

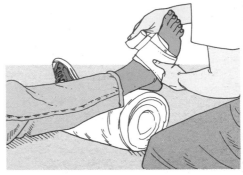

4 Control bleeding and dress any wounds, if present.

3 Raise and support his foot on a folded blanket or coat.

5 Arrange removal to hospital, keeping the foot raised and supported.

JAW & FACIAL FRACTURES

Fractures and wounds to the jaw and face may be further complicated by damage to the brain, skull, and/or bones in the neck. The main danger to the casualty is choking because the airway may be obstructed by displaced or lacerated tissues, or broken or detached teeth. He or she may be unable to swallow adequately to keep the airway clear.

LOWER JAW FRACTURES

This is usually the result of direct force, e.g., a heavy blow to the jaw. However, a blow to one side of the jaw can cause a fracture on the other side. Usually only one side of the jaw is affected but a fall on to the point of the chin can lead to a fracture of both sides.

SYMPTOMS & SIGNS
- Pain, increased by jaw movement or swallowing.
- Difficulty in speaking and may feel sick.
- Casualty may dribble because of difficulty in swallowing. Saliva is normally stained by blood issuing from tooth sockets or other mouth wound.
- Wound inside the casualty's mouth.
- Swelling, tenderness and later bruising of the casualty's face and lower jaw.
- Irregularity may be felt along the jaw.
- Irregularity of the teeth may be seen.

AIM
Maintain breathing and arrange urgent removal to hospital.

TREATMENT

1 Maintain the casualty's breathing by ensuring a clear airway.

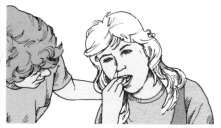

2 Control any bleeding and treat any wounds (see p.72).

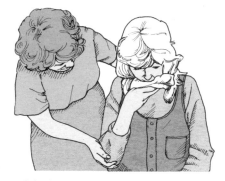

3 If she is conscious and not seriously injured, sit her up with her head well forward to allow any secretions to drain away. Support her jaw with a soft pad. Ask her to hold it in place.

4 If she vomits, support her jaw and head. Gently clean out her mouth.

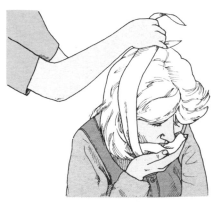

5 If her jaw is hanging down out of line, support it with a pad under the chin and bandage around her head. Tie the knot on top of her head.

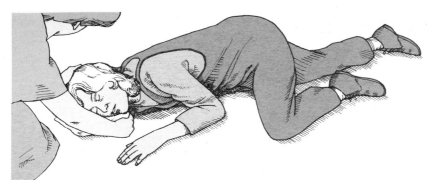

6 If the casualty has serious jaw injuries, or becomes unconscious and is breathing, place her in the Recovery Position (see p.24). *Do not apply a jaw bandage.* Place a soft pad under the casualty's head to raise it slightly to keep the weight off the jaw.

7 Carry out the ABC of Resuscitation if required (see pp.14–25); you may need to use Mouth-to-Nose Ventilation.

8 Arrange urgent removal to hospital, maintaining the treatment position.

CHEEK-BONE & UPPER JAW FRACTURES

A casualty with a cheek-bone and upper jaw fracture may be bleeding from the nose. Severe swelling of the face and bruising around the eyes may develop rapidly. The major hazard of upper jaw fractures is an obstructed airway.

TREATMENT

1 Place a cold compress (see p.173) over the injury to lessen swelling, bleeding and pain. The casualty may hold it herself.

2 Treat any mouth wound.

3 If the casualty has serious facial injuries or becomes unconscious and is breathing, place her in the Recovery Position (see p.24).

4 Arrange removal to hospital.

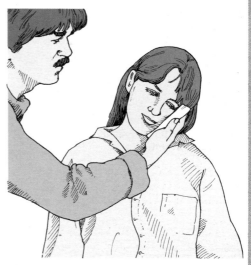

NASAL FRACTURES

Besides bleeding, the main problem associated with a nasal fracture is blockage of the airway, so every effort must be made to ensure that the casualty has an open airway. A cold compress may provide some relief (see p.173).

Treat any nose-bleed (see p.71) and remove the casualty to hospital.

BACK INJURIES

Possible injuries to the spine include fractures, displaced intervertebral discs, strains and sprains. Fractures or disc lesions may involve nerve damage. If you have any doubt about the nature of the injury, it *must* be treated as a fracture. *Always* suspect a fracture if the casualty has a history of spinal injury.

Any disturbance of feeling or movement, however slight or however temporary, should raise the possibility of a spinal fracture or spinal cord injury. The major pointer to a diagnosis is your suspicion of a fracture because of the particular circumstances of the accident.

The spine

Made up of a series of small bones or "vertebrae", the spine forms a canal through which the spinal cord runs (see p.93). Almost all vertebrae are separated by a pad of cartilage called an inter-vertebral disc. The vertebrae have limited movement upon these discs, which act as a form of "shock-absorber" in case the spinal column is jarred. The whole column of bones is supported by numerous strong ligaments and the muscles of the trunk.

The spinal cord consists of nerve fibres which run from the brain and control many of the functions of the body. It is very delicate, and damage to it can result in loss of power or sensation in all parts of the body below the injured area. Temporary damage can occur if the cord is pinched by displaced discs or bone fragments; permanent damage will occur if the cord is partially or completely severed.

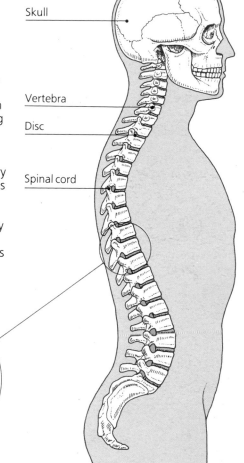

Skull

Vertebra

Disc

Spinal cord

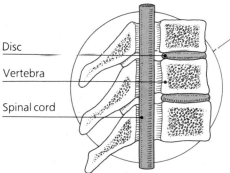

Disc

Vertebra

Spinal cord

SPINAL FRACTURES

A fractured spine is always classed as a serious injury, necessitating the greatest care in handling because it may be complicated by damage to the spinal cord.

Injury can result from both direct and indirect force. Impact from vehicle collisions and from heavy objects falling across the casualty's back, or severe jarring of the spine by falling on to the feet, buttocks or head can all result in serious spinal injury.

"Whiplash" results from the violent forward and backward movement of a person's head which commonly occurs when a vehicle is run into from behind. With this type of neck injury there may be severe ligament, muscular or nerve damage or, occasionally, the neck may be broken.

The two most vulnerable areas of the spinal column are the bones in the neck and the lower back.

SYMPTOMS & SIGNS
- Casualty may complain of severe pain in the back and may feel "cut in half".
- Casualty may have no control over limbs; ask him or her to move wrists, ankles, fingers and toes. Movements may be weak or absent.
- Possible loss of sensation. Test by gently touching limbs without the casualty's knowledge and ask if anything can be felt. Abnormal feeling, e.g., tingling, may be present.

AIM
Prevent further damage to the spine or spinal cord. Arrange urgent removal to hospital.

GENERAL TREATMENT
1 Follow the ABC rule (see p.10) – airway, breathing and circulation take priority. The positioning of the casualty depends on these priorities.

NOTE
Lifting and transporting a casualty with a suspected fractured spine is not a first-aid skill except in extreme circumstances.

DO NOT move the casualty on grounds of convenience – wait for the ambulance.

2 Maintain the position in which the casualty was found unless danger, or the priorities of airway, breathing and circulation dictate otherwise.

IF the casualty is in danger, remove him as best you can (the spine will have to take second priority, see p.165).

3 If the casualty is unconscious, open the airway by jaw lift or, if this is unsuccessful, by slight head tilt (see p.97). Clear his airway if necessary.

4 Check breathing and give Mouth-to-Mouth Ventilation if necessary (see p.18).

5 Check circulation (see p.17), and give External Chest Compression if necessary, first placing the casualty on his back by a log roll (see p.96).

6 Complete the ABC of Resuscitation by placing him in the Spinal Injury Recovery Position (see p.96).

DO NOT wait; use whatever help is available.

7 If vomiting is likely to occur and the casualty is conscious, place him in the Spinal Injury Recovery Position (see p.96) and sweep around in his mouth if necessary.

8 Steady and support the casualty's head and neck by placing your hands over his ears (do not use traction). Continue support until help arrives; while the casualty is on a stretcher; during transport to ambulance; in the ambulance until arrival at hospital.

9 If the injury is in the neck, apply a neck (cervical) collar for further support if desired (see p.127). This is *not* a substitute for support by the hands.

TREATMENT FOR FRACTURE OF BACK (CONSCIOUS CASUALTY)

1 Reassure the casualty and tell her not to move.

2 If removal to hospital is imminent, *do not move the casualty* – treat her in the position found, if possible (see p.125).

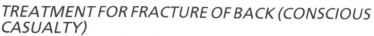

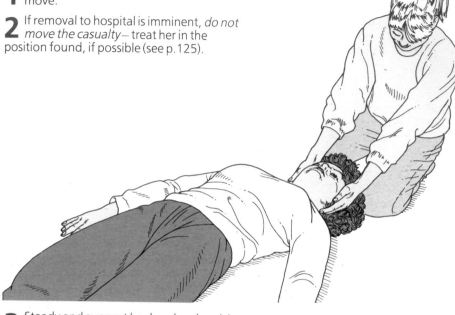

3 Steady and support her head and neck in the normal neutral position by placing your hands over her ears.

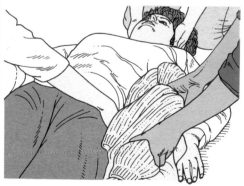

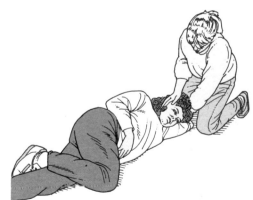

4 If helpers are available, ask them to support her shoulders and hips. Place rolled blankets or clothing alongside her trunk to give added support.

5 Cover her with a blanket, continue reassurance, and await the arrival of medical or ambulance aid.

IF vomiting is likely to occur and the casualty is conscious, place her in the Spinal Injury Recovery Position (see p.96) and sweep around in her mouth if necessary.

6 If removal from the scene is necessary, use a Scoop stretcher (see p.194).

7 If no Scoop stretcher is available, see *Manual Lift for a Fractured Spine*, p.202.

TREATMENT FOR FRACTURE OF NECK (CONSCIOUS CASUALTY)

1 Reassure the casualty and tell him not to move.

2 If removal to hospital is imminent, steady and support his head and neck in the normal neutral position by placing your hands over his ears.

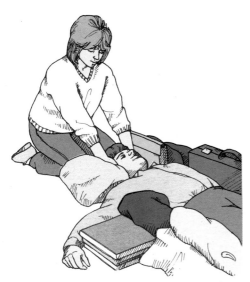

3 Place rolled blankets or other articles around his head and shoulders to give added support.

4 Cover with a blanket, continue reassurance, and await the arrival of medical or ambulance aid.

5 If removal is delayed, loosen clothing at the casualty's neck and fit a neck (cervical) collar (see right) for added stability.

NOTE
Avoid movement of the casualty's neck when fitting the collar. Continue support of his head and neck with your hands, even after the collar is fitted.

6 If the casualty must be moved, follow the procedure for a fractured back (see opposite).

FITTING A COLLAR
This may be applied to give added stability, but is *not* a substitute for support by hands.

1 If a collar is not available, fold a newspaper to a width of about 10 cm (4 in).

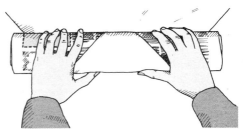

2 Wrap it in a triangular bandage or scarf, or insert it into a stocking or leg of a pair of tights. Bend it over your thigh.

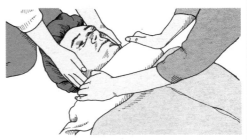

3 Place the centre of the collar at the front of the casualty's neck below the chin.

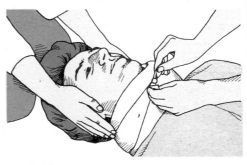

4 Fold the collar around his neck and tie in position at the front.

5 Ensure there is no obstruction to breathing.

OTHER PAINFUL DISORDERS OF THE SPINE

The most mobile parts of the spinal column are in the lower back and the neck, and these are the most common sites of muscle strain or sprain of the ligaments. In these areas, damage to the intervertebral discs (known as prolapsed or "slipped" discs) sometimes causes irritation or pressure on the adjoining nerve roots or spinal cord.

Back and neck strain may occur after prolonged bending, e.g., when gardening; with sudden lifting from a stooped position; or as a result of a "whiplash" injury (see p.125).

Other causes of backache include kidney disease and menstrual disorders.

SYMPTOMS & SIGNS
■ Dull or severe pain in the lower back (lumbago) or in the neck.
■ Possible local tenderness.
■ A spasm of the muscles may occur so that the spine is held rigidly and any attempt at bending is extremely painful.
■ Pain may pass down the back of a thigh to the lower leg (sciatica), sometimes accompanied by tingling or numbness; if the neck is affected, these symptoms may be felt down the upper limbs.

AIM
Relieve pain and seek medical aid if necessary.

TREATMENT
1 Lay the casualty down in the most comfortable position, either on the ground or on a firm mattress, until the pain eases.

2 If he has severe neck pain, fit a neck (cervical) collar (see p.127) to give relief.

3 If the symptoms persist, seek medical aid.

DO NOT lift objects with a bent back and straight knees.

DO NOT remain stooping or bending with straightened legs for lengthy periods.

DO NOT attempt to lift too heavy a weight by yourself.

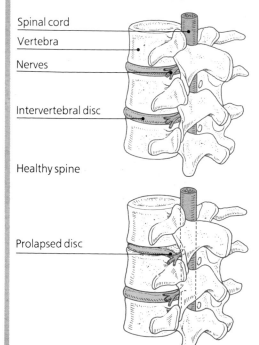

Spinal cord
Vertebra
Nerves
Intervertebral disc

Healthy spine

Prolapsed disc

Damage to an intervertebral disc
In a healthy spine, the discs separate the vertebra and cushion them. When one of the discs is damaged, it becomes distorted and presses against the nerves coming from the spinal cord.

MUSCLE & JOINT INJURIES

Injuries involving damage to the muscles, joints or ligaments which strengthen the joints are common and they can be painful. A dislocated joint in particular may also be mistaken for, or accompanied by, a fracture. In all cases where you are in doubt about an injury, treat it as a fracture and transport the casualty to hospital as quickly as possible.

How muscles work

Muscles cause the various parts of the body to move and are of two types: voluntary and involuntary; both produce movement by contracting and relaxing.
Voluntary muscles are so-called because they are under the control of the will. Their movement is co-ordinated through the motor nerves which pass directly from the brain or via the spinal cord (see p.93). The bones of the skeleton act as a framework for these muscles to pull against and the muscles are attached to the bones by bands of strong, fibrous tissue called *tendons.* Voluntary muscles operate in groups: one group contracts in order to move a bone, at the same time as its paired group of muscles relaxes so that movement can take place.
Involuntary muscles operate the vital organs, such as the heart and intestines, and work all the time, even when we sleep. Most of these muscles cannot be controlled by the will but only by the nerves in the autonomic system (see p.93).

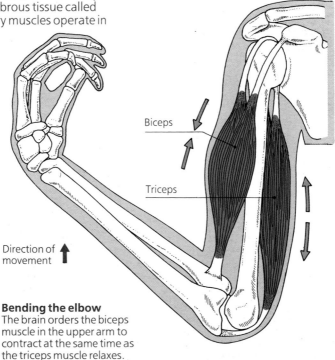

Biceps

Triceps

Direction of movement ↑

Bending the elbow
The brain orders the biceps muscle in the upper arm to contract at the same time as the triceps muscle relaxes.

STRAIN

A strain occurs when a muscle or group of muscles is over-stretched and possibly torn, by violent or sudden movement. Strain can be caused by lifting heavy weights incorrectly or when participating in sports.

SYMPTOMS & SIGNS
■ Sudden, sharp pain and/or tenderness at the injury site, which may radiate outwards with subsequent stiffness and/or cramp.
■ Swelling may develop at the site of injury.

AIM
Make the casualty as comfortable as possible and seek medical aid.

TREATMENT
This is abbreviated as **RICE: R** for *Rest*, **I** for *Ice*, **C** for *Compression*, **E** for *Elevation*.

1 Rest the injured part in the most comfortable position.

2 Apply an ice bag or cold water compress for at least 30 minutes if the strain is of recent origin (see p.173).

3 Compress the injured part by surrounding the muscle with a thick layer of cotton wool and securing it with a firm bandage to counteract swelling.

4 Elevate the injured limb.

IF you are in any doubt about the casualty's condition, treat her injury as a fracture (see pp.106–123).

5 Arrange removal to hospital.

HERNIA

An abdominal hernia or rupture is a protrusion caused by a part of the contents of the abdomen protruding through the muscular wall under the skin. A hernia may happen after exercise, while lifting heavy objects or when coughing. It occurs most frequently in the groin (1) but it is not uncommon at the navel (2) or through the scar of an abdominal operation (3).

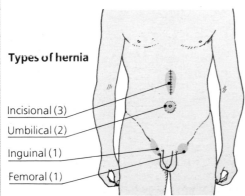

Types of hernia

Incisional (3)
Umbilical (2)
Inguinal (1)
Femoral (1)

SYMPTOMS & SIGNS
■ Painless swelling which may persist or worsen or there may be sudden, painful swelling with possible vomiting. (The latter may indicate a "strangulated" hernia, where swelling cuts off the blood supply. This condition requires urgent medical attention.)

AIM
Seek medical aid.

TREATMENT
1 Reassure the casualty.

2 Lay him down in a half-sitting position, supporting his head and shoulders. Bend his knees and support him in this position.

3 Seek medical aid urgently if the hernia is "strangulated".

DO NOT attempt to reduce the swelling.

CRAMP

This is a sudden, involuntary and painful contraction of a muscle or group of muscles. It can occur if there is poor muscular co-ordination during exercise; if chilling occurs following or during exercise such as swimming; if the body loses excessive amounts of salt and body fluids through severe sweating, diarrhoea or persistent vomiting; or during sleep. Cramps due to salt and water loss may also be associated with heat exhaustion (see p.149).

SYMPTOMS & SIGNS
■ Pain in the affected area.
■ Feeling of tightness or spasm in the affected muscles.

AIM
Relax contracted muscles and relieve pain.

TREATMENT
This condition is normally relieved by stretching the muscles. First straighten the affected part of the body, then gently massage it.

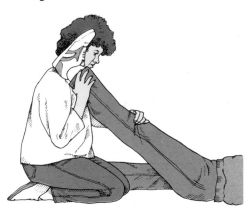

FOR CRAMP IN THIGH MUSCLES
For back of thigh, straighten the casualty's knee and raise his leg with one hand under his heel; with your other hand, press down the knee. Gently massage the affected muscles. For front of thigh, bend the knee.

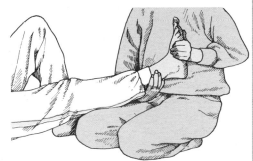

FOR CRAMP IN CALF MUSCLES
Straighten the casualty's knee and gently draw her foot upwards towards the shin. Gently massage the affected muscles.

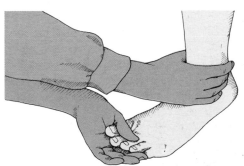

FOR CRAMP IN FOOT MUSCLES
Straighten out the casualty's toes and help her to stand on the ball of her foot. Gently massage the foot.

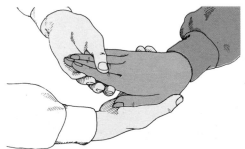

FOR CRAMP IN HAND MUSCLES
Gently, but firmly, straighten out the fingers and gently massage the area.

How joints work

Joints are formed by the junction of two or more bones and are of two types: immovable and movable.

Immovable joints are those where the bone edges fit firmly into each other or are fused together so that no movement can take place. The best example of this type of joint is in the skull.

Movable joints either allow free movement in all directions (ball-and-socket joints), movement in one plane only (hinge joints) or slightly gliding movement (slightly movable joints).

The ends of any bones forming a joint are covered in a smooth cartilage to minimize friction, and the joint is held together by bands of strong tissue called *ligaments*. The joint itself is enclosed in a capsule filled with a lubricant called synovial fluid.

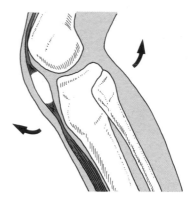

Hinge joints
When the surfaces of the bones are moulded together they only allow movement in one direction – bending (flexion) and straightening (extension). Examples are the elbow and knee joints.

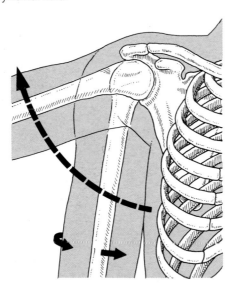

Ball-and-socket joints
Formed by the round head of one bone fitting into the cup-shaped cavity of another, ball-and-socket joints allow movement in all directions. Examples are the shoulder and hip joints.

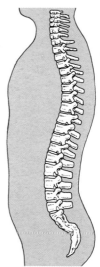

Slightly movable joints
With this type of joint only limited movement is possible. Examples are the joints between the vertebrae and those between the ribs and the spine.

SPRAIN

This injury occurs at a joint when the ligaments and tissues around that particular joint are suddenly wrenched or torn. For example, if you turn your foot over unexpectedly while walking or running you may suffer a sprained ankle. Some sprains are minor, others are associated with extensive damage to the tissues and are difficult to distinguish from fractures. In all doubtful cases, treat the injury as a fracture.

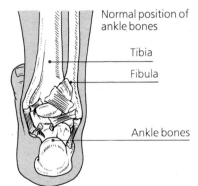

Normal position of ankle bones

Tibia

Fibula

Ankle bones

Sprained ankle
When a ligament is damaged, the ankle bones become displaced.

Wrenched ligament

SYMPTOMS & SIGNS
■ Pain and tenderness around the joint increased by movement.
■ Swelling around the joint followed later by bruising.

AIM
Make the casualty as comfortable as possible and seek medical aid.

TREATMENT
Follow the **RICE** procedure (see p.130).

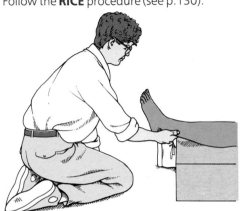

1 Rest, steady and immobilize the injured part in the most comfortable position for the casualty.

2 Carefully expose the joint and, if the sprain is of recent origin, apply an ice bag or cold water compress (see p.173) to reduce swelling, bruising and pain.

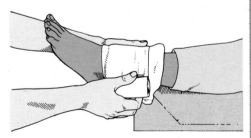

3 Help counteract swelling and provide some support by surrounding the joint with a thick layer of cotton wool; secure with a bandage.

4 Elevate the injured part.

5 Seek medical aid.

IF in any doubt about the injury, treat it as a fracture (see pp.106–123).

DISLOCATION

The displacement of one or more bones at a joint is known as "dislocation". It occurs when a strong force acts directly or indirectly on a joint, wrenching a bone into an abnormal position. Alternatively, it can be the result of a sudden muscular contraction.

Joints which are most frequently dislocated are the shoulder, thumb, finger and jaw. In some cases it is difficult or even impossible to distinguish between a dislocation and a fracture and both may be present. If in doubt, *always* treat the injury as a fracture.

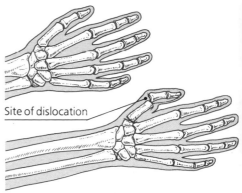

Site of dislocation

Dislocation of the thumb

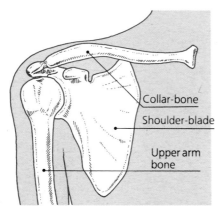

Collar-bone

Shoulder-blade

Upper arm bone

SYMPTOMS & SIGNS

■ Casualty complains of severe (often sickening) pain at or near the joint.
■ Casualty is unable to move affected part; joint "fixed" in position.
■ Injured joint appears deformed.
■ Swelling and later bruising at the site of the injury.

AIM

Make the casualty as comfortable as possible and arrange removal to hospital.

TREATMENT

1 Sit the casualty down, and support the injured part in the most comfortable position, using cushions. The casualty may be best able to support the injured part himself.

2 Immobilize with padding, bandages or slings if practical and appropriate.

3 Arrange urgent removal to hospital.

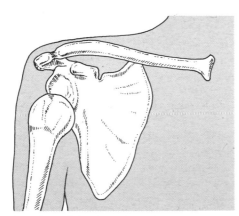

Dislocation of the shoulder
This occurs when the round end of the upper arm bone slips out of the "socket", the shoulder-blade.

DO NOT attempt to replace bones in their normal positions as further damage to surrounding tissues, blood vessels and nerves may result. If in any doubt about the injury, treat it as a fracture (see pp. 106–123).

BURNS & SCALDS

These are injuries caused by extremes of temperature (heat or cold), chemicals or radiation. Burns caused by "wet" heat such as steam or hot liquids are called scalds. For practical purposes the management of burns and scalds is the same.

Burns vary in depth, size and severity and may damage the underlying parts of the body as well as the skin. Most burns will require medical attention.

Heat is the most common cause of burns. Other causes include contact with dry or liquid corrosive chemicals, and over-exposure to radiation and sun rays.

There is considerable risk of infection with burns because the damaged skin offers reduced protection against germs. There is also a danger of shock developing, because serum (tissue fluid) leaks out of the circulatory system into the burnt area (see p.86).

TYPES OF BURN

Burns can be categorized according to the cause of the injury.

Dry burns
Flames, lighted cigarettes and hot electrical equipment such as irons are all common causes of dry burns. Fast-moving objects rubbed against the skin produce dry friction burns. Alternatively, they may be caused by the skin rubbing against an object. The most common example of this is a "rope burn".

Scalds
Wet heat such as steam, hot water or fat produces scalds.

Cold burns
These may result from contact with metals in freezing conditions. Freezing agents such as liquid oxygen and liquid nitrogen can also cause cold burns.

Chemical burns
Acids and alkalis, found in domestic cleaning products as well as in industry, may cause burns if in contact with the skin.

Electrical burns
Electrical currents and lightning generate heat and burn skin and underlying tissues.

Radiation burns
Sun rays and light reflected from a bright surface, (e.g., snow) can cause damage to the skin and eyes.

Very rarely, radiation burns can be caused by overexposure to X-rays or radioactive substances.

CLASSIFICATION OF BURNS

Burns are classified according to the area and depth of the injury. These factors determine what treatment is required and whether a casualty needs hospital attention. However, any casualty with burns covering an area greater than 2–3 cm (1 in) diameter, or burns deeper than the surface of the skin, or burns arising from electrical contact, must be referred to a doctor or hospital.

AREA
The area of a burn gives a rough guide as to whether or not a casualty is likely to suffer shock. The greater the area involved, the greater the possibility of shock, because of greater fluid loss. For example, an otherwise fit adult casualty with a superficial burn covering nine per cent or more of the body's surface will need hospital treatment.

DEPTH OF BURNS

There are three levels of burning: superficial, intermediate and deep or full-thickness burns. However, it is often difficult to distinguish between the different levels, particularly in the early stages. A large burn will almost certainly contain areas of all three.

> **NOTE**
> The severity of a burn depends upon both the area it covers and its depth.

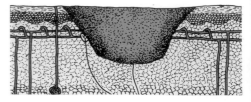

Deep burns

These burns involve all layers of skin. The skin may appear pale, waxy and sometimes charred. Because the nerve-endings are damaged, these burns are relatively pain-free. Deep burns *always* require medical attention.

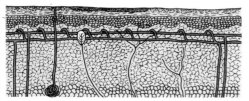

Superficial burns

These burns involve only the outer layers of skin and result in general redness, swelling and extreme tenderness. This type of burn usually heals well.

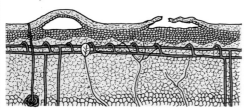

Intermediate burns

These burns involve the formation of blisters, which may be intact or broken, with an area of surrounding redness. Intermediate burns may become infected so you should seek medical aid.

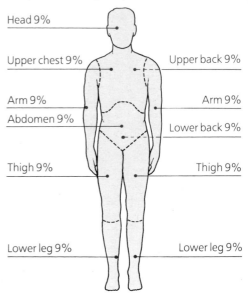

Head 9%
Upper chest 9%　　Upper back 9%
Arm 9%　　Arm 9%
Abdomen 9%　　Lower back 9%
Thigh 9%　　Thigh 9%
Lower leg 9%　　Lower leg 9%

The rule of nines

This diagram divides the body surface into areas of nine per cent. Any injury of an equivalent area will require hospital treatment. Any burn larger than 2–3 cm (1 in) diameter requires medical attention.

BLISTERS

Blisters are thin "bubbles" which form on skin damaged by friction or heat. They are caused by tissue fluid (serum) leaking into the burnt area under the surface of the skin.

During healing, new skin forms at the base of the blister underneath the serum, the serum is reabsorbed and, eventually, the outer layer of skin peels off. Never break a blister; you will increase the risk of infection.

Unless a blister breaks or is likely to be further damaged, it requires no treatment. If it does need protection, apply a dressing large enough to extend well beyond the edges of the burnt area.

CLOTHING ON FIRE

Clothing may be set on fire by standing too close to an electric fire or by carelessness in the kitchen. Without prompt help the result is widespread severe burning, shock and possible death. If the accident occurs indoors, prevent a conscious casualty from panicking and rushing outside; the movement and/or breeze outside would fan the flames.

You should lay the casualty down with the burning side up as soon as possible to prevent flames sweeping upwards, and

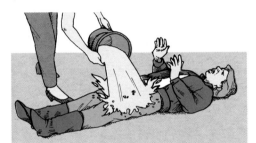

quickly put out the flames by dousing the casualty with water or other *non-flammable* liquid. Alternatively, wrap the casualty tightly in a coat, curtain, blanket (not the cellular type), rug or other heavy fabric, then lay him or her flat on the ground. This starves the flames of oxygen and puts them out.

DO NOT use nylon or other inflammable materials to smother the flames.

DO NOT roll the casualty along the ground as this can cause burning of previously unharmed areas.

IF your own clothes catch fire and help is not immediately available, extinguish the flames by wrapping yourself up tightly in suitable material and lying down.

DRY BURNS & SCALDS

These are the most common types of burns both in the home and in industry and they are a major cause of accidental death, particularly amongst children and the elderly.

Burns and scalds must be cooled as soon as possible in order to prevent further damage to underlying tissues and to alleviate pain, swelling and the possibility of shock. The most effective method of cooling is to flood the area gently with cold water.

Any clothing which has been soaked in boiling fluid should be removed as soon as it begins to cool. Cooled, dry, burnt clothing should not be removed because doing so may introduce an infection.

Very small burns or scalds can generally be treated on site. However, if you are in any doubt about the severity of the injury, or if the casualty is an infant or a sick or elderly person, always seek medical advice.

Friction burns, e.g., rope burns, should be treated as minor burns unless the skin is broken. If the skin is broken, see *Minor External Bleeding*, p.65.

GENERAL SÝMPTOMS & SIGNS
■ Severe pain in and around the injured area.
■ Redness and possible swelling of the area, and sometimes peeling of the skin and blisters, which may be broken.
■ In deeper burns the skin may appear grey, pale or waxy, or may be charred. There may be areas of numbness.
■ Symptoms and signs of shock (see p.86), which may be delayed. The degree of shock will relate directly to the extent of the injury.

AIM
Reduce the effect of the heat, prevent infection, relieve pain and minimize shock. Arrange urgent removal to hospital if burns are severe or extensive.

GENERAL TREATMENT

Treatment of burns and scalds depends on the severity of the injury.

FOR MINOR BURNS & SCALDS

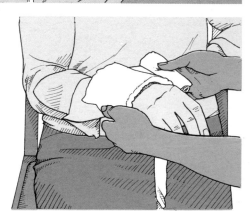

1 Reassure the casualty. Place the injured part under slowly running cold water or immerse it in cold water for *at least* 10 minutes — longer if the pain persists because the heat may not have been sufficiently withdrawn from the burnt area causing the tissues to continue to "cook".

IF no water is available, use any cold, harmless liquid such as milk or beer instead.

3 Dress the area with clean, preferably sterile, non-fluffy material (see *Dressings*, pp.169–172).

DO NOT break blisters, remove any loose skin or otherwise interfere with the injured area.

DO NOT apply lotions, ointments or fat to the injury.

DO NOT use adhesive dressings.

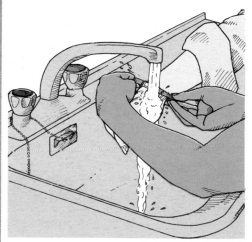

2 Gently remove any rings, watches, belts, shoes or other constricting clothing from the injured area *before* it starts to swell.

4 If in doubt about the severity of the injury, seek medical aid.

138

FOR SEVERE BURNS & SCALDS

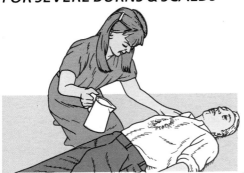

DO NOT break blisters, remove any loose skin or otherwise interfere with the injured area.

DO NOT apply lotions, ointments or fat to the injury.

1 Lay the casualty down. Protect the burnt area from contact with the ground, if possible. If the burnt area is still hot, carefully pour jugs of cold water or suitable cold liquid over the burnt area, and continue until the pain has stopped.

2 Gently remove any rings, watches, belts or constricting clothing from the injured area *before* it starts to swell.

3 Carefully remove any clothing soaked in boiling fluid after it has begun to cool.

DO NOT remove anything that is sticking to a burn.

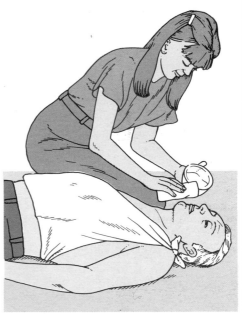

5 For facial burns indoors, cool with water until pain is relieved. No cover is usually required. Alternatively, make a mask from a clean, dry, preferably sterile piece of material (a pillow case is useful) with holes for the nose, mouth and eyes.

6 Immobilize a badly burned limb (see *Fractures*, pp.106–123).

7 To minimize shock, treat as on p.86.

8 If the casualty become unconscious, open his airway and check breathing. Complete the ABC of Resuscitation and place him in the Recovery Position (see pp.14–25).

9 Arrange urgent removal to hospital, maintaining the treatment position. Transport as a stretcher case if necessary.

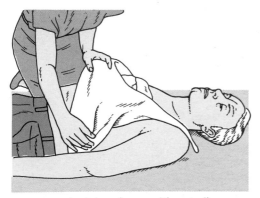

4 Cover the injured area with a sterile dressing or similar non-fluffy material, e.g., a freshly laundered sheet or pillow slip. A clean, preferably new, plastic bag may be used for an injured hand or foot. Secure with a bandage (see *Dressings*, pp.169–172).

BURNS IN THE MOUTH & THROAT

Burns to the mouth and throat usually result from drinking very hot liquid, swallowing corrosive chemicals or inhaling very hot air. These injuries are very serious because the tissues in the throat swell quickly and can close the airway making it difficult, if not impossible, for the casualty to breathe. As a result there is a real danger of asphyxia (see p.42). In this situation it is particularly important to prevent the casualty panicking, thereby worsening the situation.

SYMPTOMS & SIGNS
■ Casualty complains of severe pain in the injured area.
■ Damaged skin around the mouth.
■ Difficulty in breathing.
■ Possible unconsciousness.
■ Symptoms and signs of shock (see p.86).

AIM
Arrange urgent removal to hospital.

TREATMENT
1 Reassure the casualty.

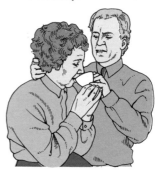

2 If she is conscious, give her sips of cold water at frequent intervals.

3 Remove any constricting clothing or jewellery from her neck and chest.

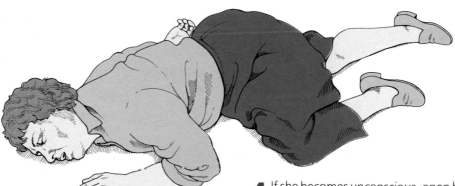

4 If she becomes unconscious, open her airway and check breathing. Complete the ABC of Resuscitation if necessary and place in the Recovery Position (see pp.14–25).

5 To minimize shock, treat as on p.86.

6 Arrange urgent removal to hospital, maintaining the treatment position. Transport as a stretcher case if necessary.

CHEMICAL BURNS

Certain substances are irritating to the skin and contact with them can cause severe damage to the tissues; eyes are particularly vulnerable. Apart from the local effects, a few chemicals may be absorbed through the skin and cause widespread and sometimes fatal damage within the body.

Strong corrosives and chemicals will be found in industry but some household goods such as caustic soda, bleaches, household cleaners and paint strippers can cause chemical burns.

While prompt action with this type of burn is important, you should *always* consider your own safety before approaching the casualty.

SYMPTOMS & SIGNS
■ Casualty may complain that skin is stinging.
■ Skin may appear stained or reddened and blistering and peeling may develop.

AIM
Identify and remove the harmful chemical as quickly as possible. Do not waste time looking for the antidote unless it is immediately available. Arrange urgent removal to hospital.

TREATMENT

NOTE
Make sure the water drains away freely and safely as it will be contaminated by the chemical which caused the burn.

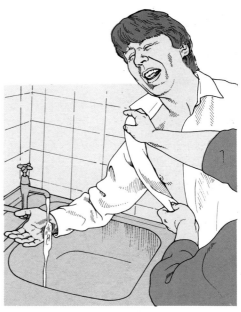

2 Gently remove any contaminated clothing while flooding the injured area; make sure you do not contaminate yourself.

3 Continue treatment for severe burns, (see p.139).

4 Arrange urgent removal to hospital; transport as a stretcher case if necessary.

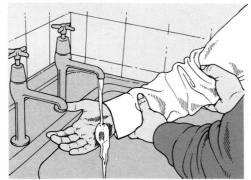

1 Flood the affected area with slowly running cold water for at least 10 minutes to prevent further damage to the burned tissues.

CHEMICAL BURNS IN THE EYE

Corrosive chemicals, both liquid and solid, can easily enter the eye and rapidly damage its surface, causing severe scarring and even blindness.

SYMPTOMS & SIGNS
- Intense pain in the affected eye.
- Damaged eye cannot tolerate light.
- Affected eye may be tightly closed.
- The eye may be reddened, swollen or watering excessively.

AIM
Wash away the chemicals as quickly as possible and arrange urgent removal to hospital.

TREATMENT

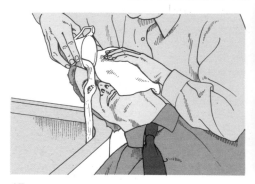

> DO NOT allow the casualty to rub his eye.

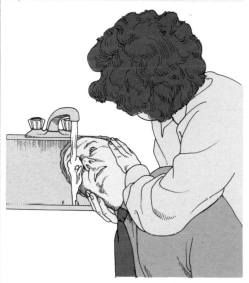

1 Hold the affected side of the casualty's face under gently running cold water so that the water drains away from his face, and not into his good eye.

IF this is not possible, sit or lay the casualty down with his head tilted back and turned towards the affected side. Protect the uninjured eye, gently open the eyelid of the affected eye and pour sterile water from an eye irrigator or a glass of tap water over it.

> NOTE
> Both surfaces of the eyelids must be well-irrigated for at least 10 minutes. If the eye is shut in a spasm of pain, pull the lids firmly, but gently, open.

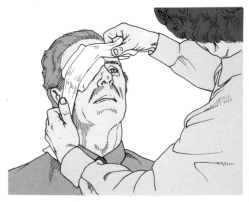

2 Lightly dress the eye with a sterile eye pad or, if this is not available, a pad of clean, non-fluffy material.

3 Arrange urgent removal to hospital.

ELECTRICAL BURNS

A burn may occur when electricity of a sufficiently high current and voltage passes through the body. Much of the damage occurs at, or close to, the points of entry and exit but, while only small burns may be visible, damage to the underlying tissues may be considerable. Electric shocks can also affect both breathing and heart action (see *Asphyxia*, p.42).

The most dangerous causes of electrical burns are high-voltage industrial machinery and lightning. Electricity in high-voltage industrial cables can jump or "arc" up to 18 m (20 yd) and kill you. So, do not approach the casualty unless you are officially informed that the current has been switched off (see p.57).

SYMPTOMS & SIGNS
■ Redness, swelling, scorching or charring of the skin at both the entry and the exit points.
■ Possible unconsciousness.
■ Breathing and heartbeat may have stopped.
■ Symptoms and signs of shock (see p.86).

AIM
Separate the casualty from the source of injury, treat the burns and arrange removal to hospital.

TREATMENT

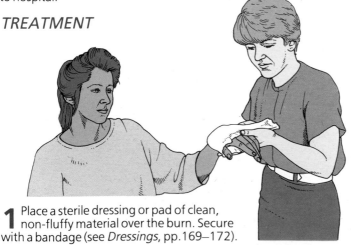

1 Place a sterile dressing or pad of clean, non-fluffy material over the burn. Secure with a bandage (see *Dressings*, pp.169–172).

DO NOT break blisters, remove any loose skin or otherwise interfere with the injured area.

DO NOT apply lotions, ointments or fat to the injury.

2 To minimize shock, treat as on p.86.

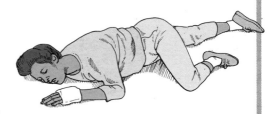

3 If the casualty becomes unconscious, open her airway and check breathing. Complete the ABC of Resuscitation if necessary and place her in the Recovery Position (see pp.14–25).

4 Arrange urgent removal to hospital, maintaining the treatment position. Transport as a stretcher case if necessary.

SUNBURN

Direct exposure to the sun's rays may produce redness, itching and tenderness of the skin. It can vary from superficial burning to a more severe reaction in which the affected skin becomes lobster-red, blistered and painful.

Overexposure to the sun's rays when it is very windy or the body is wet with sea-water or sweat can result in serious burns. However, sunburn can also occur even on a dull, overcast day in summer and in winter on high mountains when skiing because of the ultraviolet light.

SYMPTOMS & SIGNS
■ Casualty's skin will be red, tender and swollen with possible blistering.
■ Affected skin will feel hot.

AIM
Remove the casualty to a cool place and seek medical aid if the burns are severe.

TREATMENT
1 Place the casualty in the shade. Cool his skin by sponging gently with cold water.

2 Treat for general effects of overheating (see p.149).

3 Give him sips of cold water at frequent intervals.

4 For extensive blistering, seek medical aid urgently.

DO NOT break blisters.

SNOW BLINDNESS, WELDER'S FLASH & RADIATION

When the eyes are exposed to glare produced by the reflection of the sun on snow or concrete for too long, the cornea of the eye can be injured. This painful condition can take as long as a week to subside. It can easily be prevented by wearing dark glasses.

This condition can also result from the ultraviolet light produced by welding. Most protective helmets and goggles give complete protection but careless use may expose the eyes to a flash from an adjacent torch.

SYMPTOMS & SIGNS
These normally appear some time after exposure to glare, welding flash or radiation.
■ Casualty complains of intense pain in the affected eyes; eyes may feel gritty.
■ Affected eyes will be red, watering and sensitive to light.

AIM
Cover the eyes and seek medical aid if injury is severe.

TREATMENT

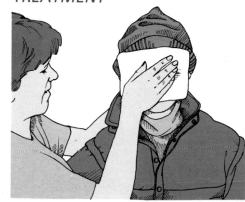

1 Bathe the eyes with cold water (see p.142).

2 Lightly dress both eyes with eye pads or similar pads of clean, non-fluffy material.

3 If in doubt about the severity of the injury, seek medical aid urgently.

EFFECTS OF EXTREMES OF TEMPERATURE

Excessive heat or excessive cold may injure the skin or deeper tissues, and in extreme cases, may so upset the working of the body that death may ensue.

Our bodies work most efficiently within a normal temperature range of 36–37° C (97–99° F). In order to keep a level temperature the body must retain heat when the environmental temperature is cold and lose heat when it becomes hot.

Body heat is under the control of a temperature control centre (''thermostat''), situated at the base of the brain, which automatically adjusts the mechanisms that keep the balance between heat loss and heat gain. Heat is lost by radiation as the small arteries and capillaries in the skin dilate, thereby increasing circulation and diverting heat from the vital organs. Heat is also lost by the cooling effect of sweating and in the vapour breathed out from the lungs. Conversely, heat is retained by shutting down these processes. Therefore when it is hot, the skin is flushed and moist; when cold, it is pale and dry. Moreover, the rate of breathing is more rapid in hot environments than in cold.

Temperature regulation may sometimes be inadequate for the circumstances and it tends to be less effective in the very young or very old.

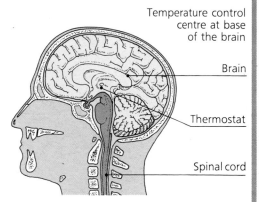

Temperature control centre at base of the brain

Brain

Thermostat

Spinal cord

THE EFFECTS OF COOLING

Body temperature tends to fall when the environmental temperature falls below a critical point – this varies according to the fitness, acclimatization or reactions of the individual. The most rapid falls are encountered when heat is lost by conduction, e.g., by immersion in a cold sea.

The body reacts to cold by constricting the small blood vessels of the skin to reduce circulation at the surface and to conserve heat at the centre of the body in order to protect vital organs. The heat at the centre of the body is known as ''core temperature''.

In addition, shivering and increased muscular activity may occur. These mechanisms are designed to increase the production of body heat. High energy food and warm drinks have the same effect.

Cold injury may be either generalized (hypothermia) or localized, particularly in the extremities of toes, fingers, nose or ears (frostbite).

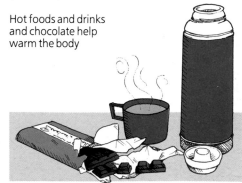

Hot foods and drinks and chocolate help warm the body

HYPOTHERMIA

This condition develops when body temperature falls below about 35° C (95° F). Moderate hypothermia can normally be reversed and recovery will be complete. However, recovery is unlikely if the body temperature falls below 26° C (75° F).

Hypothermia is commonly caused by exposure to extreme cold on mountain-sides or on moors, especially if the cold is accompanied by rain, mist or snow, or by immersion in cold seas, lakes or rivers. Wind-chilling also increases the danger.

Hypothermia may also be encountered in poorly heated houses, particularly in elderly people and infants. Lack of physical fitness, fatigue, hunger and dehydration increase the risk of hypothermia. Thin people are more readily affected than fat.

PREVENTION

In order to lessen the dangers of suffering from hypothermia outdoors, you must plan and train for expeditions carefully. No one suffering from minor illness should take part. Choose several layers of loose clothing with an outer waterproof layer. Clothes should be loose at the neck and wrists to allow evaporation of sweat after exercise. Carry spare, dry socks, and keep sleeping bags dry and aired. Take high energy foods, and never smoke or drink alcohol.

To prevent hypothermia in the home, provide adequate heating and bedclothes.

SYMPTOMS & SIGNS

The onset of hypothermia may be insidious and difficult to recognize.
■ Casualty may be shivering if in the early stages of hypothermia.
■ Casualty's skin is cold, pale and dry.
■ Casualty's temperature is subnormal – 35° C (95° F) or less.
■ Casualty may behave irrationally and gradually slip into unconsciousness.

■ Pulse and respiratory rates are slower than normal.
■ As the casualty becomes unconscious, breathing and pulse become increasingly difficult to detect and the heart may stop and require resuscitation.

AIM

Prevent casualty losing any more body heat, and help to regain normal body temperature.

TREATMENT

NOTE
Never presume that the casualty is dead simply because you cannot detect breathing or a pulse.

IF CASUALTY IS AT HOME OR IN SHELTER

1 Remove the casualty's outer clothing, and replace any wet clothing with dry.

2 Place her in a bed which has been previously warmed.

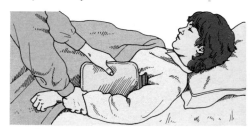

3 Place a suitably covered hot-water bottle in her left armpit or over her breastbone (this warms the "core" circulation).

DO NOT place hot water bottles at her extremities as this increases blood flow through the limbs, which are still cold, and may result in a dangerous fall in "core temperature".

4 To rewarm her more quickly, place her in a hot bath, at a temperature which is bearable when tested with your elbow (approximately 43° C/110° F). Test the water at intervals, and replenish if necessary. When the casualty's skin colour returns to normal and her pulse rate improves, return her to a warm bed.

5 Give her hot drinks and high energy food, e.g., chocolate.

NOTE
It is best to rewarm victims of hypothermia at the speed at which cooling took place. A person rescued after falling into the sea should be rewarmed rapidly. An elderly person, or infant, who has slowly become hypothermic overnight, should be rewarmed gradually.

IF CASUALTY IS IN THE OPEN

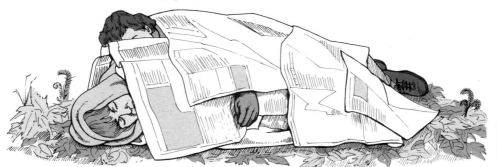

1 Carry the casualty to a warm shelter as quickly and as gently as possible. Insulate the ground she is to lie on, e.g., with dry bracken.

2 Place her in a sleeping bag or cover her with blankets, newspaper, silver foil, or other insulating materials.

3 Whilst awaiting rescue, lie beside the casualty so that you share your body heat with her.

4 Send for help (ideally, you should send two people).

5 When help arrives, evacuate the casualty by stretcher to hospital or to a house to await the ambulance or helicopter.

IF she is conscious, give her hot drinks and high energy food.

IF she is unconscious, open her airway and check breathing. Complete the ABC of Resuscitation if necessary, and place her in the Recovery Position (see pp. 14–25).

HYPOTHERMIA IN INFANTS
Babies can suffer from hypothermia as they have difficulty in regulating their body temperatures. A baby with hypothermia may look very healthy so that its behaviour may be the only indication. Rewarm gradually and seek urgent medical aid.

SYMPTOMS & SIGNS
■ The baby is unusually quiet, drowsy and limp.
■ The baby will refuse food.
■ Usually, the face, hands and feet are bright pink and healthy looking.

HYPOTHERMIA IN THE ELDERLY
In addition to being less able to regulate their body temperatures, the elderly and the infirm are often unable to look after themselves – they go without adequate food and heat and may not feel like moving about. In the aged, hypothermia may be mistaken for a stroke or heart attack. Rewarm gradually and seek urgent medical aid.

FROSTBITE

This is a condition in which local tissues are frozen, usually at the extremities. They become injured by prolonged constriction of the surface blood vessels as a result of exposure to extreme cold. As with heat burns (see p.135), the damage may be either superficial or deep, and the affected tissues may be destroyed.

To prevent frostbite, wear adequate clothing and gloves, and leave as little skin exposed as possible.

SYMPTOMS & SIGNS

■ The affected areas – tip of nose, ears, fingers or toes – become at first pale, then waxy white, later a mottled blue colour, and finally black.
■ Blistering may occur.
■ Casualty may complain of "pins and needles" and intense pain, but the part gradually becomes numb and pain disappears as the freezing bites deeper.
■ The skin feels hard and stiff.

AIM

Warm the affected area *slowly* and naturally to prevent further tissue destruction. Arrange removal to hospital.

TREATMENT

NOTE
If there are signs of accompanying hypothermia (see p.146), treat this before frostbite.

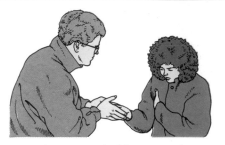

1 At first signs of whiteness, pain or tingling, handle damaged tissues gently. Remove frozen coverings carefully, together with rings or watches. Warm the part with your own hands. Alternatively, if a finger is frostbitten, place the casualty's affected hand in her opposite armpit until normal colour returns.

2 Get her to warm surroundings as soon as possible. She may walk on frostbitten feet before thawing-out, but *never* afterwards – carry her on a stretcher.

IF colour does not return rapidly, place the affected part in warm water (tested first with your elbow).

3 As the part thaws out, the colour will improve and pain will return. Dry and dress the thawed area with dry gauze or wool and lightly bandage it.

4 Elevate the limb to reduce swelling.

5 If authorized by a doctor, give the casualty two paracetamol tablets.

6 Arrange removal to hospital, transport as a stretcher case.

DO NOT attempt to thaw-out a part if the casualty will later be exposed to cold or a journey, as to freeze-thaw-refreeze is disastrous for tissues. Simply cover the affected part in dry gauze, wool and loose bandaging, or enclose it in a plastic bag.

DO NOT rub the area.

DO NOT burst blisters.

DO NOT heat the part with fires or hot-water bottles.

DO NOT allow the casualty to smoke.

THE EFFECTS OF OVERHEATING

During strenuous exercise, heat is released in the muscles and distributed to all parts of the body by the blood, causing the general body temperature to rise. When this happens, the body reacts immediately to lose heat.
■ The skin capillaries enlarge (dilate), so that more blood is carried to the surface, allowing heat to be lost by radiation. This diversion of blood to the skin makes the person look hot and flushed.
■ The sweat glands produce more sweat, which evaporates and cools the body.
■ Breathing increases and more heat is lost from the lungs.

Two conditions can arise from overheating – heat exhaustion and heatstroke. *Heat exhaustion* usually affects people performing physical exercise in hot, moist environments, especially if they do not replace the fluid and salt lost in sweat.
Heatstroke and rapid unconsciousness can occur during exposure to extreme heat or high humidity where there is no air current. The body temperature may rise as high as 43° C (110° F) because of the affected person's inability to sweat.

HEAT EXHAUSTION

This condition is caused by loss of salt and water from the body. It is more common in persons unaccustomed to working in a very hot, humid environment, although in elderly persons it may follow a debilitating illness. Heat exhaustion can be aggravated by a stomach upset with diarrhoea and vomiting.

SYMPTOMS & SIGNS
■ Casualty may feel exhausted but restless.
■ Casualty may have a headache and feel tired, dizzy and nauseated.
■ Muscular cramps may occur in abdomen and lower limbs, caused by salt deficiency.
■ Casualty's face will be pale and the skin will feel cold and clammy.
■ Breathing becomes fast and shallow.
■ Pulse is rapid and weak.
■ Temperature may remain normal or fall.
■ Casualty may faint on sudden movement.

AIM
Remove the casualty to a cooler environment and replace lost fluids and minerals. Seek medical aid.

TREATMENT
1 Lay the casualty down in a cool place.

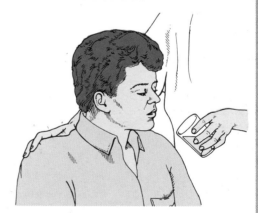

2 If he is conscious, give him sips of cold water to drink.

IF he is sweating profusely, has cramps, diarrhoea and/or is vomiting, add half a teaspoon of salt to each ½ litre (1 pint) of water.

3 If the casualty becomes unconscious, open his airway and check breathing. Complete the ABC of Resuscitation if necessary, and place him in the Recovery Position (see pp. 14–25).

4 Seek medical aid.

HEATSTROKE

This is caused by a very high environmental temperature or a feverish illness, such as malaria, that leads to a greatly raised body temperature. It develops when the body can no longer control its temperature by sweating and can occur quite suddenly. It can develop in people of any age who have been exposed to heat and high humidity for too long and who are unaccustomed to them. It can also be caused by prolonged confinement in a hot atmosphere. Anyone suffering from heatstroke should always receive urgent medical attention.

SYMPTOMS & SIGNS
■ Casualty complains of headache, dizziness and of feeling hot.
■ Casualty becomes restless.
■ Unconsciousness may develop rapidly and may become very deep.
■ Casualty is hot with a temperature of 40° C (104° F) or more and will look flushed although his or her skin remains dry.
■ Pulse is full and bounding; breathing may be noisy.

AIM
Reduce the casualty's temperature as quickly as possible and seek medical aid.

TREATMENT
1 Move the casualty to a cool environment and remove her clothing.

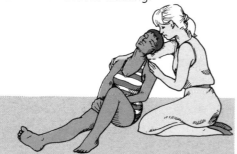

2 If she is conscious, place her in a half-sitting position with her head and shoulders supported.

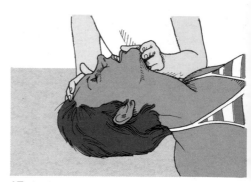

IF she is unconscious, open her airway and check breathing. Complete the ABC of Resuscitation if necessary, and place her in the Recovery Position (see pp. 14–25).

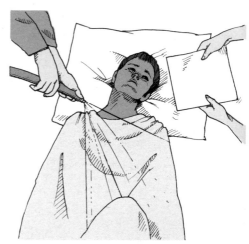

3 Wrap her in a cold, wet sheet and keep it wet. Direct currents of air on to her by fanning with a magazine or an electric fan until her temperature falls to 38° C (101° F).

4 Seek medical aid immediately.

IF her temperature falls, cover her with a dry sheet and remove her to an air-conditioned room if possible.

IF her temperature rises again, repeat steps 3 and 4 above.

POISONING

A poison is any substance that, if taken into the body in sufficient quantity, can cause temporary or permanent damage. Instances of alleged poisoning occur in the United Kingdom each year involving both children and adults and some of them are fatal. Whilst some cases are attempted suicides, others are accidental and involve substances in everyday use. Whatever the cause of poisoning, medical aid should always be sought as soon as possible. *Never* attempt to make the casualty vomit; it is ineffective and you may worsen the situation.

The digestive system

Food is broken down in the mouth, stomach and intestines by digestive juices secreted by various glands. It is taken in at the mouth and travels down the gullet (oesophagus) until it reaches the stomach. After partial digestion in the stomach, food then passes into the small intestine in small amounts. Here it is broken down into simple substances which are absorbed by the blood. The residue, consisting largely of vegetable fibres, enters the large intestine where accompanying water and mineral salts are absorbed. The final waste products are then eliminated from the body through the rectum at the anus.

The liver acts as a chemical factory which, amongst other functions, inactivates some poisons. The kidneys rid the blood of many impurities.

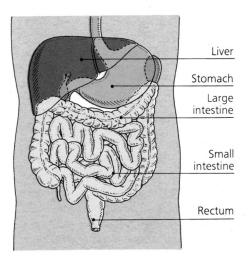

Liver
Stomach
Large intestine
Small intestine
Rectum

HOW POISONS ENTER THE BODY

Poisons can enter the casualty's body in a number of ways either accidentally or intentionally:
■ Through the mouth by eating or drinking poisonous substances.
■ Through the lungs by inhaling household or industrial gases (not North Sea gas; it is not poisonous), chemical vapours, or fumes from fires, stoves, faulty appliances and petrol-engine exhausts.
■ By injection into the skin as the result of bites from some animals, insects, poisonous fish or reptiles or by hypodermic syringe.
■ By absorption through the skin through contact with poisonous sprays such as pesticides and insecticides.

HOW POISONS ACT

When in the body poisons act in various ways. Once in the bloodstream, some poisons work on the central nervous system preventing breathing, heart action and other vital processes. Other poisons act by displacing the oxygen in the blood and preventing its distribution to the tissues.

Swallowed (ingested) poisons also react directly on the food passages, resulting in vomiting, pain and often diarrhoea. Corrosive poisons may severely burn the lips, mouth, gullet and stomach, thus causing intense pain.

GENERAL SYMPTOMS & SIGNS

These vary depending on the nature of the poison and the method of entry into the body.
■ Information from the casualty or an onlooker suggesting contact with a poison. Try to ascertain exactly what was involved and, if swallowed, when and how much was taken.
■ Presence of a container near the casualty known to hold or have held poison or a poisonous plant.
■ Casualty may be delirious and have convulsions (without previous history of such conditions).
■ Symptoms and signs of asphyxia (see p.42).
■ Unconsciousness may develop.
■ If the poison was swallowed, the casualty may begin retching or vomiting or suffer from diarrhoea.
■ Burns around the casualty's mouth after contact with corrosive poisons.

NOTE
A casualty attempting suicide may dispose of any evidence which would aid diagnosis.

AIM
Maintain an open airway, breathing and circulation and get the casualty to medical aid or hospital as soon as possible.

GENERAL TREATMENT

1 Quickly ask the conscious casualty what has happened; remember that he may lose consciousness at any time.

DO NOT attempt to induce vomiting.

IF his lips or mouth show signs of burning, cool them by giving him water or milk to sip slowly.

2 Place him in the Recovery Position (see p.24) even if he is not unconscious (he may vomit).

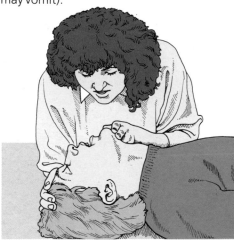

3 If consciousness is lost, follow the ABC of Resuscitation immediately (see pp.14–25).

NOTE
Take care not to contaminate yourself with any poison that may be around the casualty's mouth.

4 Arrange urgent removal to hospital. Send with him any samples of vomit and any containers such as bottles or pill boxes found nearby.

HOUSEHOLD POISONS

Many substances found in and about the home can be poisonous. These include liquid soap, some cosmetics, fire-lighters, white spirit, bleach, glue, rat-poison, paint stripper, garden sprays and insecticides. Children are especially at risk from such materials since they may not or cannot be aware of the consequences of eating or drinking them.

The symptoms and signs will vary according to the poison, although vomiting and abdominal pain are likely to occur in most cases. Treat the casualty as described on p.152 and remove to hospital.

Children are also liable to take medicines and tablets found in medicine cabinets.

While most household medicines and tablets are not dangerous if taken as directed, many are poisonous if the dosage is exceeded. Some of the more dangerous medicines include capsules and tablets which look like sweets, especially the coloured ones, e.g., certain iron tablets, tranquillizers and barbiturates.

NOTE
Always make sure that all bottles and jars containing poisonous substances are clearly marked and kept out of reach of children.

Potentially poisonous substances in the home
Medicines, household cleaning materials and garden insecticides can all be dangerous if eaten or drunk, especially by children.

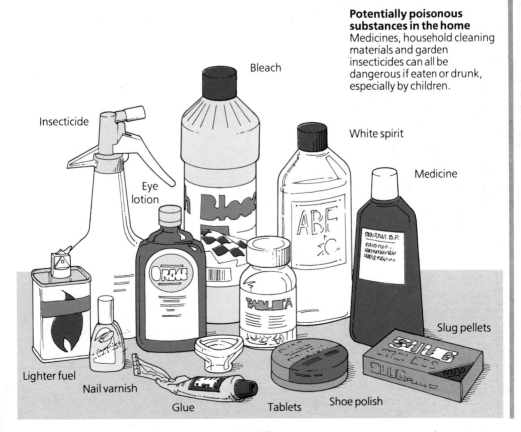

Bleach

Insecticide

Eye lotion

White spirit

Medicine

Slug pellets

Lighter fuel

Nail varnish

Glue

Tablets

Shoe polish

POISONOUS PLANTS

Certain plants, around our gardens as well as in the wild, are dangerous if eaten and some may cause allergic reactions if touched. Children, in particular, are attracted by the bright berries of many of these plants and sometimes eat them.

Laburnum (Laburnum anagyroides), deadly nightshade (Atropa belladonna) and death cap fungus (Amanita phalloides) are the more common examples of plants which can poison the system. The symptoms and signs of this type of poisoning are similar to those of food poisoning (see below). The severity of the condition will depend upon how much of the plant has been taken. If you suspect that a casualty has eaten a poisonous plant or berries, it is important that you maintain an open airway and remove the casualty to hospital immediately.

There are very few plants in the United Kingdom which cause a reaction when touched. However, contact with those that are likely to cause a reaction, e.g., nettles, may result in a mild rash or swollen eyelids.

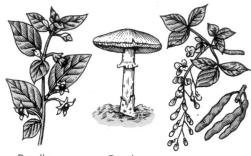

Deadly nightshade   Death cap fungus   Laburnum

FOOD POISONING

This is caused by food becoming contaminated by bacteria and being stored or cooked incorrectly. The most common bacteria are: *staphylococci*, which multiply in the food and produce a poisonous substance (toxin); or *salmonellae*, which multiply in the bowel and cause a dysentery-like illness. Salmonella is infectious and can be passed through poor personal and kitchen hygiene.

SYMPTOMS & SIGNS
These depend upon the type of poisoning.

Staphylococcal poisoning
These symptoms and signs will appear within two to six hours of eating contaminated food.
- Casualty will feel nauseated and may already be vomiting.
- Casualty may be suffering from abdominal pain and may have a headache.
- Diarrhoea may develop at a later stage.
- Symptoms and signs of shock (see p.86).

Salmonella poisoning
The symptoms and signs of salmonella poisoning may appear within a few hours of eating or be delayed for a day or two.
- Casualty develops a fever.
- Casualty will be suffering from diarrhoea.
- Casualty may feel nauseated and vomit.
- Casualty may have abdominal pain.
- Symptoms and signs of shock (see p.86).

AIM
Seek medical aid.

TREATMENT
1 Follow the general treatment for poisoning.

2 Make sure the casualty rests.

3 Give him plenty of fluids to drink.

4 If in doubt, arrange removal to hospital.

DRUG POISONING

This condition is caused by an accidental overdose or drug abuse. Drug abuse may be broadly defined as the self-administration of a drug in a manner that is not in accordance with approved medical or social patterns. Drugs can be inhaled, swallowed or injected into the body. A regular drug abuser may show signs of continuous use of hypodermic injections. These marks will usually be on the front of the forearm near the elbow, although other places are used. The veins in the area will become inflamed and infected.

Drugs commonly abused are: narcotics (e.g., heroin); depressants (e.g., barbiturates and tranquillizers); stimulants (e.g., amphetamines); and hallucinogens (e.g., L.S.D.). In addition, there is solvent inhalation (e.g., "glue-sniffing").

SYMPTOMS & SIGNS
These will vary according to the drug and the quantity taken. Vomiting will not always appear immediately but you should watch for it. The pupils of the eyes may be abnormally dilated or contracted.

Narcotics
These are usually injected but can be taken in tablet form or inhaled.
- Breathing becomes difficult and eventually will cease.
- Casualty may have injection marks on the front of one or both arms.

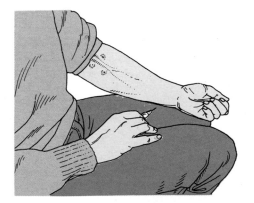

Depressants
- Breathing will be shallow.
- Casualty's skin will feel cold and clammy.
- Pulse will be weak and rapid.
- Possible unconsciousness.

Stimulants
- Casualty will be excitable and sweating profusely.
- Casualty may be suffering from tremors and hallucinations.

Hallucinogens
- Casualty will be anxious and sweating.
- Casualty may be behaving strangely and suffering from hallucination.

Aspirin overdose

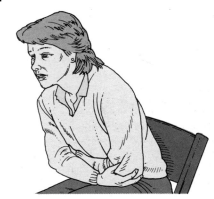

- Casualty has abdominal pain, and may be vomiting. Vomit may be blood-stained.
- Casualty may be depressed and drowsy.
- Casualty may complain of "ringing" in the ears (tinnitus).
- Difficulty in breathing.
- Casualty will be sweating profusely.
- Pulse will be full.

TREATMENT
1 Follow the general treatment for poisoning.

2 Arrange urgent removal to hospital and be prepared to resuscitate.

ALCOHOL POISONING

Alcohol is a drug that depresses the central nervous system. It affects different people in different ways. One drink usually only produces a slight change in mood. As the intake continues, however, the drug affects the areas of higher reasoning within the brain – those that control restraint and judgement. As the concentration of alcohol in the blood increases, the behaviour of the drinker becomes exaggerated and co-ordination will be impaired. Eventually, the mental and physical abilities are deeply disturbed and unconsciousness will develop.

SYMPTOMS & SIGNS
■ Casualty's breath may smell of alcohol.
■ Casualty may be vomiting.
■ Casualty may be partly conscious or already unconscious. If unconscious you may be able to rouse him or her, but he or she will lapse into unconsciousness again quite quickly.
In early stages of unconsciousness:
■ Casualty will be breathing deeply.
■ Face will be moist and flushed.
■ Pulse will be full and bounding.
In later stages of unconsciousness:
■ Pulse may become rapid but weak.
■ Breathing will be shallow.
■ Casualty's face will feel dry and look bloated.

■ Eyes will be bloodshot and pupils may be dilated.

NOTE
If there is a head injury it may alter the symptoms and signs (see pp.69 and 98–101).

AIM
Ensure an open airway; arrange removal to hospital if the casualty is unconscious.

TREATMENT

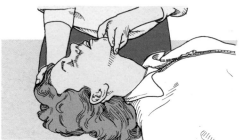

1 Maintain an open airway (see p.14).

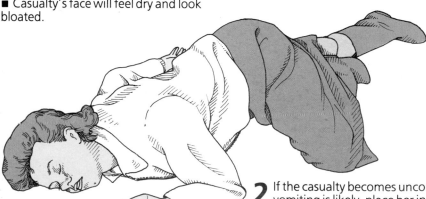

2 If the casualty becomes unconscious or vomiting is likely, place her in the Recovery Position. Complete the ABC of Resuscitation if necessary (see pp.14–25).

3 If in doubt about her condition, arrange removal to hospital.

INDUSTRIAL POISONS

Some people may be in contact with dangerous chemicals or gases at their workplaces as a result of the failure of a chemical plant, for instance, or spillage of corrosive substances.

Amongst the most common industrial poisons are gases. These are usually classed as: irritants (e.g., ammonia and nitrous fumes); asphyxiants (e.g., carbon dioxide); toxic gases (e.g., carbon monoxide and hydrogen cyanide gas); and toxic vapours (e.g., those given off by volatile chemicals such as carbon-tetrachloride or trichloroethylene).

There are so many different poisonous substances in use that it is impossible to give a comprehensive list. Any factory using potentially dangerous chemicals or gases must display notices indicating any special action to be taken in case of accidents (see *Accidents Involving Dangerous Substances*, p.168). Therefore, if you are called to an industrial accident involving dangerous substances, contact a responsible works official. Always obey any safety regulations to avoid further injury to both yourself and the casualty.

Remember that any casualty suffering from the effects of gas or toxic fumes needs air. Take great care to prevent yourself being overcome by any fumes that remain in the area. Never attempt to rescue a casualty trapped in an enclosed space unless you are equipped with, and practised in the use of, breathing apparatus and life-lines.

ANAPHYLACTIC SHOCK

This condition is a massive allergic reaction which can develop within a few seconds or minutes of an injection of a drug or insect sting to which the casualty is sensitive. More rarely it follows the ingestion of an allergen such as penicillin, in which case the reaction will be slower.

SYMPTOMS & SIGNS

■ Symptoms and signs of shock (see p.86).
■ Casualty will feel nauseated and may be vomiting.
■ Casualty complains that chest feels tight.
■ Difficulty in breathing – casualty may be wheezing and gasping for air.
■ Casualty may be sneezing.
■ There may be facial swelling especially around the eyes.
■ Pulse will be rapid.
■ Unconsciousness may develop.

AIM

Arrange urgent removal to hospital and be prepared to resuscitate.

TREATMENT

1 Follow treatment for shock (see p.86).

2 Maintain an open airway. If the casualty's breathing becomes difficult, place the casualty in the Recovery Position (see p.24).

3 If the casualty becomes unconscious, complete the ABC of Resuscitation (see pp.14–25).

4 Arrange urgent removal to hospital.

FOREIGN BODIES

A "foreign body" means any extraneous matter that enters the body either through a wound in the skin (penetrating) or via one of the natural openings of the body (inserted or swallowed), or that enters the eye.

A penetrating foreign body can be anything that enters the body, from a tiny splinter of wood or glass to a large wooden stake or piece of metal. It may be loose and easily removed without causing further pain or injury or it can be embedded. The latter may, in addition, be acting as a plug preventing blood loss (see p.64).

Large embedded foreign bodies may produce a deep wound but small splinters cause little more than minor lacerations.

The main problem with injuries involving penetrating foreign bodies is that foreign bodies are rarely clean so there is a high risk of infection (see *Infected Wounds*, p.68).

SPLINTERS

Wood and metal splinters which have become embedded in the skin are probably the most common foreign bodies. They can generally be removed with tweezers as described below. However, if the splinter is deeply embedded or over a joint, seek medical aid as soon as possible.

SYMPTOMS & SIGNS
■ Known contact with pieces of wood, metal or glass.
■ An embedded foreign body may be visible.
■ Pain and tenderness in the area.

AIM
Gently remove the splinter.

TREATMENT
1 If the area around the splinter is dirty, cleanse it using soap and water (see *Minor External Bleeding*, p.65).

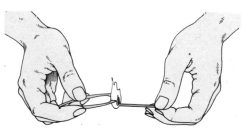

2 Sterilize a pair of tweezers by passing them through a flame.

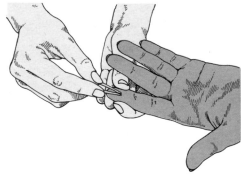

3 Gently try to pull the splinter out of the wound with tweezers. Hold the tweezers as near to the skin as possible and grasp the splinter; pull the splinter out in the opposite direction to that in which it entered the skin.

4 If the splinter does not come out easily or begins to break up, treat as an embedded foreign body (see p.64) and seek medical aid.

DO NOT probe the area to reach the splinter.

NOTE
Make sure the casualty's tetanus inoculation is up-to-date (see p.68).

FOREIGN BODIES IN THE EYE

All eye injuries are potentially serious because particles may perforate the eyeball resulting in internal damage, possible infection and blindness.

Particles of dust or grit or loose eyelashes are the most common foreign bodies found in the eyes. They stick to the outer surface of the eyelid, normally the upper lid, causing considerable discomfort and inflammation. In most cases these can easily be removed. However, *never* attempt to remove a foreign body if it is on the coloured part of the eye (pupil and iris) or embedded in the eyeball; seek medical aid immediately.

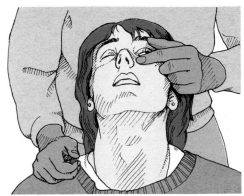

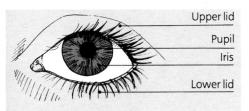

Upper lid
Pupil
Iris
Lower lid

SYMPTOMS & SIGNS
- Casualty's eye is painful and itches.
- Casualty's vision may be impaired.
- Watering of affected eye.
- Casualty's eye is red.

AIM
Remove particle gently. If unsuccessful, remove casualty to hospital.

TREATMENT
IF the foreign body is on the coloured part of the eye or it is embedded in or sticking to the eyeball, *do not attempt to remove it.* Advise the casualty not to move her eye. Cover it with an eye pad. If necessary, prevent eye movement by covering both eyes. Arrange removal to hospital. For treatment of chemicals in the eye, see p.142.

1 Advise the casualty *not* to rub her eye (she will almost certainly be doing so).

2 Ask her to sit down in a chair facing the light and lean back.

3 Stand behind her with her head resting against you. Use the index finger and thumb of one hand to separate the affected lids. Ask her to look right, left, up and down so that you can examine every part of the eye.

4 If you can see the foreign body try to wash it out with a *sterile water solution* and an eye irrigator. If these are not available, irrigate the eye with tap water. Incline the casualty's head towards the injured side so that the water will drain out over her cheek away from the sound eye; pour water from a jug or place her head under a tap.

5 If this is unsuccessful or no water is available and the foreign body is *not* sticking to the casualty's eye, lift the foreign body off using a moistened swab or the damp corner of a clean handkerchief.

6 If the foreign body is under her upper lid, ask her to look down. Grasp the eyelashes and pull the upper lid downwards and outwards over *the lower lid*. If the lashes of the lower lid do not brush the foreign body off, get the casualty to blink the eye under water in the hope that it will float off.

7 If you cannot remove the foreign body, cover the affected eye with an eye pad or a piece of gauze wrapped around a soft pad of cotton wool. Secure it lightly in position and seek medical aid.

FOREIGN BODIES IN THE NOSE

These are usually encountered in very young children who try to insert various objects such as pebbles or marbles into their noses. Smooth objects may just be lodged in the nose but a sharp object can easily damage the tissues of the nose. Do not attempt to remove the object but remove the casualty to hospital.

SYMPTOMS & SIGNS
- Casualty has difficulty in breathing through the nose.
- The nose may be swollen.
- Discharge (often blood-stained) appearing from one or both sides of the nose.

AIM
Reassure the casualty and arrange removal to hospital as soon as possible.

TREATMENT
1 Keep the casualty quiet and advise him to breathe through his mouth.

2 Arrange removal to hospital.

> **DO NOT** attempt to remove the foreign body.

FOREIGN BODIES IN THE EAR

These are most common in children. They can cause temporary deafnesss but deep penetration can damage the eardrum. Alternatively, insects may become lodged in the ear.

SYMPTOMS & SIGNS
- Casualty may complain of pain in the ear.
- Casualty may feel vibrations if an insect is inside the ear.
- Hearing on the affected side may be impaired.

AIM
Arrange removal to hospital.

TREATMENT
1 Reassure the casualty.

2 If a foreign body is suspected, *do not* attempt to dislodge it as probing may perforate the eardrum.

3 If it is an insect, sit the casualty down with the affected ear uppermost, and place a towel over his shoulder.

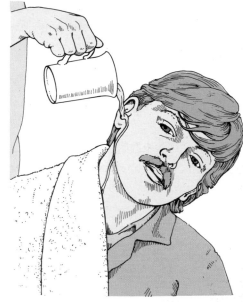

4 Gently flood the casualty's ear with tepid water so that the insect will float out.

5 Arrange removal to hospital, if necessary.

INSECT STINGS

Insects, such as bees, wasps and hornets, or jellyfish such as Portugese-Men-of-War cause stings which are more painful and alarming than they are dangerous. Some people, however, are allergic to the poison. Moreover, multiple stings from a swarm of insects can have a dangerous cumulative effect (see *Anaphylactic Shock*, p.157). Stings in the mouth and throat may cause swelling leading to asphyxia (see p.42).

SYMPTOMS & SIGNS
■ Unexpected sharp pain; an insect may still be present.
■ There will be swelling around the affected area with a central reddened puncture point.
■ Possibility of shock depending on the degree of reaction (see p.86).

AIM
Remove sting if present and attempt to reduce swelling and relieve pain. If the sting is inside the mouth, arrange urgent removal to hospital.

TREATMENT
FOR STINGS IN THE SKIN

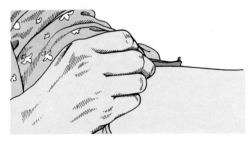

1 If the sting has been left embedded in the skin, hold the tweezers as near to the skin as possible, grasp the sting and remove it (see p.158).

DO NOT squeeze the poison sac because this will force the remaining poison into the skin.

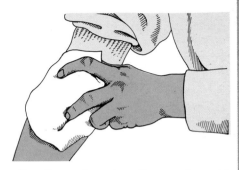

2 To relieve pain and swelling, apply a cold compress (see p.173), surgical spirit or a solution of bicarbonate of soda. For jellyfish stings, smooth calamine lotion into the affected area.

3 If pain and swelling persist or increase over the next day or so, advise the casualty to seek medical aid.

FOR STINGS IN THE MOUTH OR THROAT

1 To reduce the swelling, give the casualty ice to suck. Alternatively, rinse his mouth with cold water or a solution of water and bicarbonate of soda, if available (one teaspoon to each tumbler).

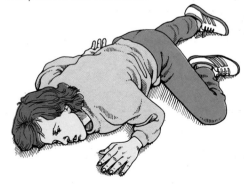

2 If breathing becomes difficult, place him in the Recovery Position (see p.24).

3 Arrange removal to hospital.

FISH HOOKS IN THE SKIN

Sometimes only the point of the hook enters the skin, in which case the hook can easily be removed. If, however, the barb is caught as well, do not try to remove it but seek medical aid. Attempt to remove it only if medical aid is not immediately available.

SYMPTOMS & SIGNS
■ Embedded fish hook may be visible.

AIM
Gently remove the point and treat as a minor wound. Seek medical aid if the barb has penetrated.

TREATMENT

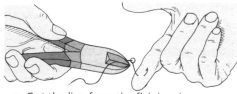

1 Cut the line from the fish hook.

2 If the barb is not caught in the skin, remove the hook and treat as a minor wound (see p.65).

3 If the barb is caught in the skin, treat as an embedded foreign body (see p.64) and seek medical aid.

IF MEDICAL AID IS NOT READILY AVAILABLE

1 Cut the line from the fish hook with a pair of pliers.

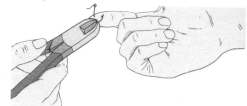

2 As long as there is no danger of damaging internal organs, push the hook through the skin until the barb protrudes, then cut through the shaft between the barb and the skin.

3 Gently withdraw the hook, clean the wound and cover with a dressing.

4 Seek medical aid to deal with any infection in the wound. A tetanus booster may be required.

SWALLOWED FOREIGN BODIES

Children in particular often swallow small objects such as pins, coins or buttons. Most small smooth objects are unlikely to damage the intestine or cause choking. However, sharp objects such as pins or needles can damage the gastro-intestinal tract (oesophagus, stomach or intestine).

SYMPTOMS & SIGNS
■ Information from the casualty or bystanders that object has been swallowed.

AIM
Reassure the casualty and arrange removal to hospital.

TREATMENT

1 Reassure the casualty and the parents if the casualty is a child.

2 Arrange removal to hospital.

DO NOT give the casualty anything by mouth.

ACHES

An ache is a continuous dull pain. Some aches are symptomatic of a condition or injury referred from another part of the body.

While it is not always possible for you to diagnose the cause of the symptoms, you should attempt to provide temporary relief from the pain. However, the administration of medicines is beyond the scope of First Aid. On the other hand, if someone suffering from a minor ache is carrying pain-killing tablets, he or she may be able to deal with the ache in this way.

Treatments for the more common aches are described on the following pages. It is important that you look for any symptoms or signs that indicate a more serious condition, e.g., chest pain may be caused by heart attack, in which case appropriate treatment described elsewhere should be given and medical aid sought immediately.

AIM
The aim of all treatment for aches is to relieve discomfort.

HEADACHE

Common causes of headache are: sinusitis, the common cold, stress, eye strain, pressure and lack of sleep or food. However, injuries to the head or spine can also result in headaches.

SYMPTOMS & SIGNS
■ Pain anywhere in the head which may be constant, throbbing or intermittent.

TREATMENT
1 Place a cold compress (see p.173) or covered hot-water bottle on the casualty's forehead, whichever is preferred.

2 Advise the casualty to take one or two of his own pain-killing tablets if available.

3 If practical, advise the casualty to lie down in a darkened room.

4 If the headache persists, or if it is accompanied by a feeling of nausea, vomiting, fever, stiff neck, disturbed vision, obvious head injury, confusion or gradual loss of consciousness, seek medical aid.

MIGRAINE

These severe and at times incapacitating headaches sometimes occur for no apparent reason and cannot normally be traced to any particular disorder. However, they may follow lack of food, noise, heat, travelling, or emotional disturbances.

Migraine attacks are more severe than normal headaches but they are not as common. The First Aider will not be able to distinguish between the two, but the treatment is the same for both conditions.

SYMPTOMS & SIGNS
■ Casualty may experience "flickering" vision – this can precede the headache.
■ Casualty will be feeling nauseated and may already be vomiting.
■ Intense throbbing headache which may only affect one side of the head.
■ Casualty cannot tolerate light or noise.
■ Casualty may look very pale.

TREATMENT
Treat as for headache, above.

TOOTHACHE

Frequent causes of toothache are decay and irritation of the gums. Pain may be referred from other structures, e.g., ears, or caused by inflammation of a facial nerve (neuralgia).

SYMPTOMS & SIGNS
■ Pain in the teeth or jaws, which may be constant, throbbing or intermittent. The pain may be made worse by cold or hot food and drink, and may vary in intensity and character.

TREATMENT
1 Carefully dab the affected tooth cavity (not the gum) with oil of cloves, if available, to deaden pain unless there is a history of sensitivity to oil of cloves.

2 Permit the casualty to take one or two of his own pain-killing tablets, if available, e.g., paracetamol.

3 Rinse his mouth with hot or cold water, whichever gives the greater relief.

4 Suggest he uses an extra pillow when lying down.

5 Advise him to visit his dentist (or doctor) at the earliest convenience even if the pain has disappeared.

EARACHE

This is often the result of an infection in or near the ear, e.g., a boil in the ear canal or a tooth abscess. The most common cause, however, particularly in children, is middle-ear infection caused by germs spreading from the throat to the middle ear. This type of infection may follow illnesses such as tonsillitis, measles or influenza. Earache can also occur when there is too much wax present in the ear canal or if there is a sudden change of pressure on the eardrum during air travel or underwater swimming.

SYMPTOMS & SIGNS
■ Constant or throbbing pain in the ear.

TREATMENT
1 To relieve a severe or persistent earache, hold a covered hot-water bottle or heated pad against the affected ear.

2 Permit the casualty to take one or two of his own pain-killing tablets, if available.

3 If earache is caused by a sudden change of pressure, advise the casualty to hold his nose and close his mouth and then swallow or blow out his cheeks.

4 If the ache persists or it is accompanied by discharge, fever, impaired hearing and/or balance, seek urgent medical aid.

ABDOMINAL PAIN

Possible causes of abdominal pain include indigestion, colic, menstrual cramp, food poisoning and constipation. Generally, it is not considered serious if it lasts less than half an hour and there are no other symptoms e.g., headache, vomiting, or diarrhoea.

SYMPTOMS & SIGNS
■ Pain anywhere in the abdomen.

TREATMENT
1 Place the casualty in the most comfortable position. Reassure him.

DO NOT give him anything by mouth.

2 If pain lasts more than half an hour, seek medical aid.

PROCEDURE AT MAJOR INCIDENTS

Major incidents are those in which a large number of casualties are involved. They can be natural, e.g., an earthquake, or involve human error, as in a road traffic accident. The number of casualties, and the sequence in which they will need to be treated, will vary according to the incident and the types of injury. Casualties may be trapped, thrown some distance or found wandering about in a dazed condition. In a major fire, injuries may be caused by people jumping out of a high building or being trapped in a smoke-filled room.

In any emergency, the way you approach the situation is important (see p.30). This is especially true in a major incident and because a single First Aider cannot treat all the casualties at once, it is essential that a brief reconnaissance of the scene is made. You will need to find out: exactly what has happened; whether danger still threatens; how many casualties there are and what condition they are in. All this information must then be passed on to the emergency services immediately (see p.32). If there is no further danger, you should then treat the casualties on site according to the priorities of airway, breathing, circulation, bleeding and unconsciousness (see p.31).

The general rule for dealing with any casualty in danger is: remove the danger from the casualty and, *only if this is not possible*, remove the casualty quickly and carefully from the danger.

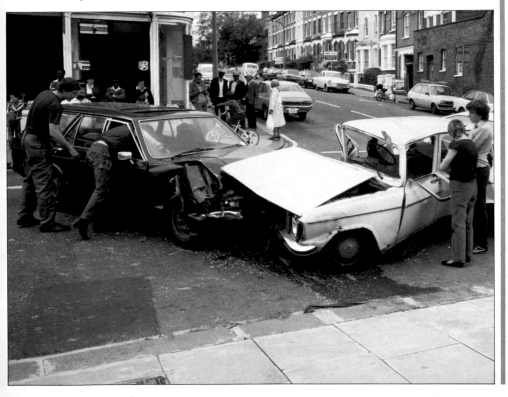

ROAD TRAFFIC ACCIDENTS

The general principles for dealing with any major incident can best be illustrated by the procedure for dealing with casualties in a road traffic accident. The most important thing to remember is that you should not put yourself at risk. Do not attempt to move a casualty unless absolutely necessary – leave it to the emergency services.

Taking calculated risks

In many road traffic accidents casualties may have to be moved in order to save lives. The decision to do so, however, should be *very* carefully considered, especially if the casualty is unconscious, because of the risk of spinal injury or severe internal bleeding.

Unless casualties are in danger of further injury, e.g., from fire, or breathing and heartbeat have stopped, you should carry out a full examination (see pp.33–36) to determine the extent of the injuries before moving them. Then, follow the procedure described below.

IMMEDIATE ACTION

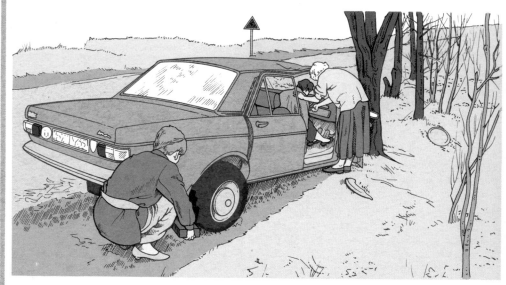

- Instruct bystanders to warn approaching traffic and set up warning triangles at least 200 m (220 yd) from the accident; if no triangles are available, ask bystanders to direct traffic.
- Look for any indication of dangerous substances being present, e.g., Hazchem warnings (see p.168).
- Instruct someone to telephone the emergency services immediately (see *Calling for Assistance*, p.32).

- Do not pull casualties from the vehicle – this could result in further injuries.
- Minimize the risk of fire by switching off the engine and, if you know how, disconnecting the battery, because fires often begin in the wiring under the bonnet or dashboard. Do not allow anyone to smoke near the vehicle. If a diesel lorry, bus or car is involved, switch off the fuel supply – there is normally an emergency switch on the outside of the vehicle.

■ Immobilize the car. If it is on four wheels, apply the handbrake, put the car into gear and/or place blocks under the wheels. If the car is on its side and there are passengers inside, *do not try to right it*, just make sure that it will not roll over.

■ Look inside the vehicle for any small children who may have fallen out of sight or be hidden under blankets or luggage. Check the area immediately surrounding the vehicle for any passengers who may have been thrown out of the vehicle or who may be wandering about. Ask a conscious casualty how many people were in the vehicle before the accident.

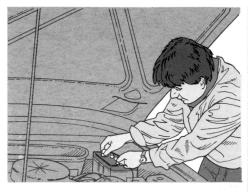
Disconnecting the battery

MOVING THE CASUALTY

If the situation is such that a casualty needs to be moved, then it must be done very carefully. He or she should be immobilized as far as possible and you should make sure that you have enough people to support all parts of the body. If bystanders are helping you, they must be given clear instructions on how the casualty is going to be moved. Each person should know exactly what he or she has to do (see *Handling & Transport*, pp.188–206) and the removal should be carried out in one continuous movement if possible.

If a casualty is trapped under a vehicle and has to be removed before the emergency services arrive, e.g., because of the danger of fire, try to move the vehicle away from the casualty first. If this is not possible, immobilize the vehicle as described left, and move the casualty as gently as possible. Remember to note the exact position of the casualty or vehicle before moving either,

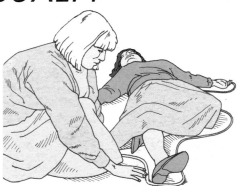
Marking the casualty's position

because the police may need this information later.

If you have decided against moving the casualty you should always be prepared to do so should the casualty's condition deteriorate or new danger threaten.

DEALING WITH TRAPPED CASUALTIES

Accident victims may be trapped in their vehicles by an impacted steering wheel for instance. Such a casualty should be watched carefully because, if unconscious, the tongue may fall to the back of the throat and block the airway. To guard against this possibility,

the casualty's head should be maintained in an open airway position (see p.14). A trapped casualty must be observed continuously until the arrival of skilled help. (See *Unconscious Casualty in a Crashed Vehicle*, p.97.)

ACCIDENTS INVOLVING DANGEROUS SUBSTANCES

Accidents may be complicated by the spillage of dangerous liquids or the escape of toxic fumes, and any such incident should be approached with great care. Never make any rescue attempt unless you are sure that you are not endangering yourself by coming into contact with a dangerous substance.

Most vehicles carrying dangerous substances now display warning notices. If you are in doubt about the meaning of the sign, keep your distance, especially if there is any spillage. Make a careful note of the code and give the information to the emergency services. Keep bystanders well away from the scene and bear in mind that poisonous fumes may be given off. If this does occur, stand upwind of the accident so that any fumes are blown away from you.

Hazard warnings
Vehicles carrying dangerous goods display hazard warning information panels indicating the substance being carried.

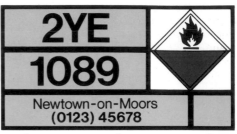

Newtown-on-Moors
(0123) 45678

Flammable
substances

Poisonous
substances

Oxidizing
agent

Radioactive
substances

Corrosive
substances

Compressed
gases

FIRES

Rapid and clear thinking is vitally important when dealing with fires. Fire spreads very quickly so warn people in the building and alert the emergency services immediately, giving them as much information as possible. Try to get everyone out of the building and make sure that all doors of rooms where there is a fire are shut. *Remember, do not attempt to fight a fire unless you have notified the emergency services and have made sure that you will not be in any danger.*

Modern furniture often contains synthetic materials which, when burning, may give off toxic fumes. So you should never enter a burning building you suspect contains poisonous fumes unless equipped with, and practised in the use of, breathing apparatus. If for any reason you do have to enter a smoke-filled room, make sure you are not endangering yourself.

If you are trapped in a burning building, the best thing to do is to go into a room with a window and shut the door. Put a blanket or carpet against the bottom of the door to keep the smoke out and call for help from the window.

If the casualty is trapped in a garage with the car engine running (see p.47), open the garage doors to ensure a good supply of fresh air. Do not attempt to enter the area until you are certain that you will not endanger yourself by doing so.

NOTE
All the above principles apply if you are involved in an incident where there is a gas leak.

DRESSINGS & BANDAGES

The type of dressings and/or bandages used and the techniques for applying them vary according to the type of injury sustained and the materials available. Dressings and bandages are sold in sterile packs. Substitutes can be made from household linen or any other clean non-fluffy material.

NOTE
Fluffy material should *never* be placed directly on to a wound because the fibres will adhere.

DRESSINGS

A dressing is a protective covering which is placed on a wound to help control bleeding, prevent infection and absorb any discharge.

All dressings should be large enough to cover the area of the wound and extend about 2.5 cm (1 in) beyond it. They should, if possible, be sterile so as not to introduce germs (bacteria) which could cause infection. A dressing should also be absorbent because, if sweat cannot evaporate, the skin around the wound will become moist and the dressing sodden. This will encourage the growth of bacteria and prevent healing.

Dressings help the blood to clot. Although a dressing may stick to a wound, making it difficult to remove, the benefits of a dressing outweigh any damage done on removal. If a dressing becomes stained by blood immediately, do not take it off, but cover it with further dressings, as necessary.

GENERAL RULES OF HYGIENE

■ If circumstances permit, wash your hands thoroughly before attending to wounds. Cover any exposed cuts or breaks in your own skin with a waterproof dressing.
■ If a wound is not too large and bleeding is under control, clean it and the surrounding skin before applying the dressing (see p.65).
■ Avoid touching the wound or any part of the dressing which will be in contact with a wound.
■ Never talk or cough over a wound or the dressing.
■ If necessary, cover non-adhesive dressings with pads of cotton wool to help control bleeding and absorb discharge. These pads should extend well beyond the dressing and be held in position by a bandage (see p.174).
■ If a dressing slips off a wound before you are able to secure it, renew the dressing – the first one may have picked up germs from the surrounding skin.

■ Always place a dressing directly on to a wound, never slide it on from the side.
■ Wash your hands with soap and water after carrying out the dressing procedure.

PLANNED FIRST AID ACTIVITIES
■ Remember that in handling a wound, blood or excreta, you yourself may be in danger of infection. Mop up spills and disinfect using one part of household bleach to 10 parts of water.
■ If you are attending a casualty who has an infection, use disposable gloves if possible.
■ Place all used dressings or infected material in a plastic bag and seal and label. Dispose by incineration.
■ Place all needles or sharp items in a sealed tin and dispose.

ADHESIVE DRESSINGS

Commonly known as "plasters", these dressings consist of an absorbent gauze or cellulose pad held in place by an adhesive backing. The best have a water-repellent adhesive backing which allows moisture to evaporate from the skin. *Waterproof* plasters should *always* be used by food handlers and, where necessary, by First Aiders. They should not be left on for more than a few hours. All plasters are supplied in sterile wrappings and they are available in a variety of shapes and sizes to fit a variety of wounds.

Always make sure the skin around a wound is clean and dry before applying an adhesive dressing; otherwise it will not stick (see p.65).

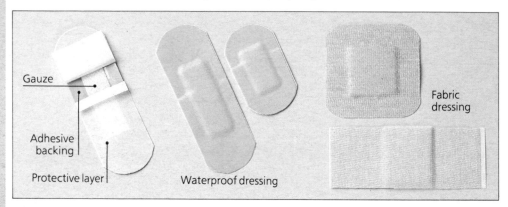

Gauze

Adhesive backing

Protective layer

Waterproof dressing

Fabric dressing

METHOD

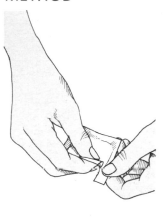

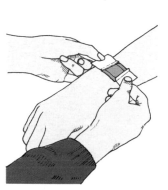

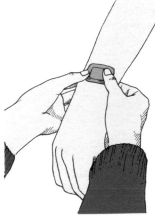

1 Remove the outer wrapping and hold the dressing, gauze-side down, by the protective strips.

2 Peel back, but do not remove, the protective strips and, without touching the gauze, place the pad on to the wound.

3 Carefully pull off the protective strips and gently press the ends and the edges down.

STERILE DRESSINGS

These consist of a dressing made up of layers of fine gauze or lint and a pad of cotton wool attached to a roller bandage.

Sterile dressings are the preferred First Aid dressings for large wounds. If available, they should be used in preference to any other type of combination dressing and/or bandage on any wound. Made in a variety of shapes and sizes, sterile dressings are always sold enclosed and sealed in protective wrappings. *Do not use a sterile dressing if the seal is broken.*

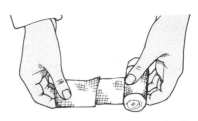

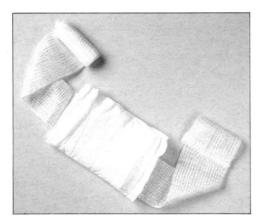

METHOD

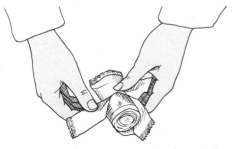

1 Remove the outer wrapping by twisting or pulling apart the outer package and remove the inner wrapping. Alternatively, pull back the tab at the end of the box and remove the inner wrapping.

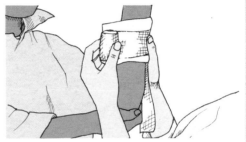

2 Holding the folded dressing and rolled bandage in one hand, unwind the short end of the bandage with the other hand.

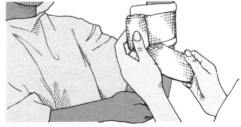

3 Hold both ends of the bandage with the folded dressing gauze-side down and over the wound; open out the dressing. Control it by placing your thumbs on the edge of the dressing (avoid touching the surface), then place it on the wound.

4 Wind the short end of the bandage once around the limb and dressing to secure it. Hold this end to the side while applying the roll. Bandage firmly until the pad is covered (see p. 183).

5 Secure the bandage by tying the ends over the pad using a reef knot (see p. 177).

GAUZE DRESSINGS

These consist of layers of gauze which form a soft, pliable covering for large wounds or burns where no sterile dressings are available. If a gauze dressing is used instead of a sterile dressing, cover the gauze with a pad of cotton wool and secure it with adhesive strapping or, if pressure is required, a bandage.

METHOD

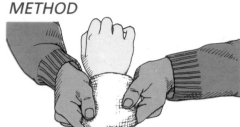

1 Remove the outer wrapping. Hold the dressing by the edges over the wound; lower it into place.

2 If necessary, cover the gauze with one or two layers of cotton wool.

3 Secure the pad with a bandage or adhesive strapping.

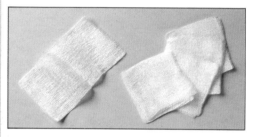

ADHESIVE STRAPPING

If bandages are not available or they are ineffective or difficult to apply, lengths of special adhesive strapping can be used to secure non-adhesive dressings to wounds. Adhesive strapping is available in a variety of lengths and widths.

NOTE
Some people have skin reactions to adhesive strapping. Inquire before applying.

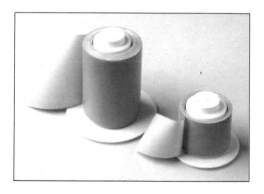

IMPROVISED DRESSINGS

In some emergencies prepared dressings may not be available. Improvise using whatever suitable materials are to hand, e.g., a clean handkerchief, a freshly laundered towel, a piece of linen or a pad of clean paper handkerchiefs can be used. Do not place cotton wool, lint, woolly or fibrous material directly on a wound; the fibres can become embedded in it.

Improvised dressings should be covered and held in position using whatever materials are available at the time, e.g., a folded scarf.

COLD COMPRESSES

Closed injuries such as bruises and sprains must be cooled to minimize swelling and relieve pain. This is best achieved by placing the injured area under cold running water. However, if the injury is on an awkward part of the body, e.g., the head or chest, or prolonged application is required, a cold compress or an ice bag may have to be used instead.

APPLYING A COLD COMPRESS

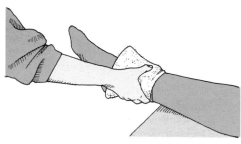

1 Soak a pad of cotton wool, towelling or similar cloth in cold or iced water. Squeeze or wring it out so that it is damp but not dripping, and place it on the injury.

2 To ensure that the cooling effect is maintained, replace the pad with a fresh compress or drip more cold water on to the old one. Continue cooling the injury for 30 minutes.

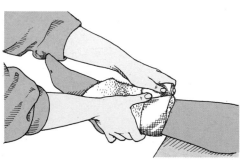

3 If necessary, cover the compress with an open-weave bandage to hold it lightly in position.

APPLYING AN ICE BAG

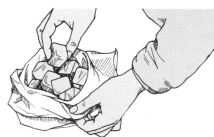

1 Fill a plastic or similar non-porous bag half to two-thirds full of crushed or cubed ice; add a little salt to lower the melting temperature of the ice. Exclude all air from the bag, seal it and wrap it in a cloth. A bag of frozen peas wrapped in a cloth may also be used.

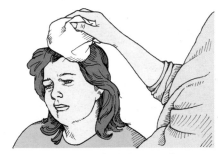

2 Place the bag over the injury; replace as necessary. Continue cooling the injury for at least 30 minutes.

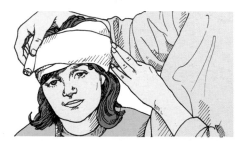

3 If necessary, cover the ice bag with an open-weave bandage to hold it in position.

BANDAGES

Bandages are used to:
■ Maintain direct pressure over a dressing in order to control bleeding.
■ Hold dressings or splints in position.
■ Prevent swelling.
■ Provide support for a limb or joint.
■ Restrict movement.
■ Occasionally, to assist in lifting or carrying casualties.
They should *not* be used for padding when other softer materials are available.

Prepared bandages are made from cotton, calico, elastic net, special paper or other materials. They are of two main types — triangular bandages and roller bandages. In an emergency, bandages can be improvised from any of the above materials or by using tights or stockings, ties, scarves or belts.

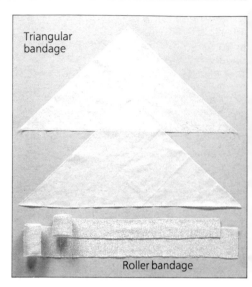

Triangular bandage

Roller bandage

GENERAL RULES FOR APPLYING BANDAGES

■ Apply bandages when a casualty is sitting or lying down.
■ Always try to sit or stand in front of the casualty and work from the injured side.
■ Before you start bandaging, make sure the injured part is well-supported in the position in which it is to remain.
■ If the casualty is lying down, pass all bandages under the natural hollows of the ankles, knees, back and neck. To ease them into position, gently pull them backwards and forwards and move them up or down the body.
■ Bandages should be firm enough to hold the dressing in position, control bleeding or prevent movement, but not so tight that they interfere with the circulation (see *Checking Circulation*, opposite).
■ Make frequent checks to ensure that the bandages are not becoming too tight as the tissues swell.

■ Where a limb is involved, expose the fingernails or toe-nails so that they can be checked for circulation (see opposite).
■ If a bandage is used to control bleeding and maintain direct pressure, tie the knot over the pad or dressing.
■ If using bandages to immobilize a limb or part of the body, tie the knots in front on the uninjured side unless otherwise specified. If both sides of the body are injured, tie the knots in the centre of the body.
■ When using a knot to secure a bandage *always* use a reef knot (see p.177).
■ Ensure there is adequate padding between the upper limbs and the body and between the lower limbs at the bony areas (e.g., the knees and ankles). Pay particular attention to filling the natural hollows (e.g., the armpits and thighs) before applying slings and bandages.

CHECKING CIRCULATION

Immediately after applying a bandage and at 10-minute intervals thereafter, it is important to check that the circulation and/or nerves have not been interfered with by the bandage. This can be checked as indicated below and, if any of the symptoms and signs are present, adjust or remove the bandage as necessary.

SYMPTOMS & SIGNS OF RESTRICTED CIRCULATION

- Casualty experiences tingling or lack of feeling in his or her fingers or toes.
- Casualty may be unable to move his or her fingers or toes.
- Casualty's finger or toe-nail beds may be pale or blue.
- Casualty's fingers or toes are very cold.
- Pulse is absent or weak in injured limb compared to that of uninjured limb.

METHOD

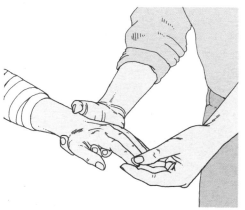

1 Press one of the nails or skin of the bandaged limb until it turns white.

2 Release pressure; the part should quickly become pink again, showing that blood has returned.

IF the nail remains white or blue or the fingers are unnaturally cold, the bandage is too tight.

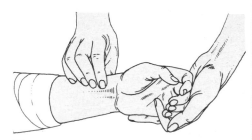

IF no radial pulse can be felt in the affected arm, the bandage is too tight.

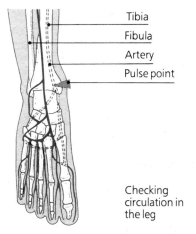

Tibia

Fibula

Artery

Pulse point

Checking circulation in the leg

Circulation in the lower limb

A pulse for the feet may be felt, with difficulty, just below and behind the lower end of the tibia at the ankle joint on the inside of either leg. This procedure requires a great deal of experience to be carried out with confidence. If the pulse can be felt, it is a useful confirmation of circulation in the foot.

NOTE

Whenever further swelling may be expected to develop, e.g., from a fracture or sprain, pad the area with rolls of soft material where possible, before applying the bandage.

TRIANGULAR BANDAGES

These can be made by cutting in half diagonally a piece of material (linen or calico) not less than 1 m (1 yd) square. Alternatively, triangular bandages can be bought, often wrapped in sterile packages.

Triangular bandages can be used in a number of ways. Open or unfolded bandages can be used to form a sling to provide support or protection for the arms or chest or for securing dressings over areas such as the head, hand and foot. Alternatively, they can be folded according to specific requirements (see opposite).

STORING TRIANGULAR BANDAGES

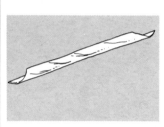 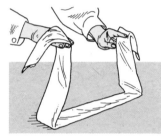 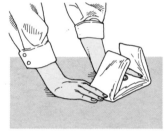

1 Make a narrow-fold bandage as in steps 1 and 2 opposite.

2 Turn the ends of the bandage into the middle.

3 Continue folding the ends into the middle until a convenient size is reached.

Parts of a triangular bandage

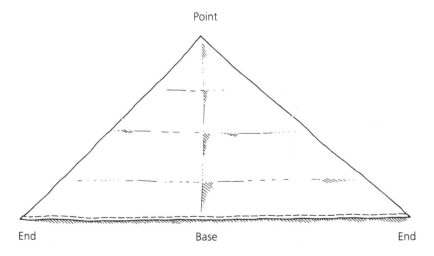

Point

End   Base   End

BROAD-FOLD BANDAGES

These folded triangular bandages are used for immobilizing limbs during transportation or for securing splints or dressings.

METHOD

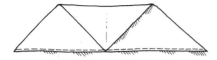

1 Turn in a narrow hem along the base of the bandage. Fold the point to the base.

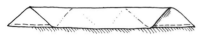

2 Fold the whole bandage in half again in the same direction.

NARROW-FOLD BANDAGES

These are useful for securing a dressing at a joint if no other bandage is available (e.g., around the ankle or wrist).

METHOD

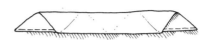

1 Make a broad-fold bandage as in steps 1 and 2, left.

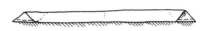

2 Fold the bandage in half again in the same direction.

REEF KNOTS

Always secure the ends of a bandage with a reef knot because it will not slip, it lies flat and is therefore more comfortable for the casualty, and it is easy to untie. Once the knot is tied, the ends should be tucked out of sight or neatly fastened to the bandage. Make sure that the knot does not press on to a bone or into the skin when used on a sling. If the knot is uncomfortable, place some soft padding under it.

METHOD

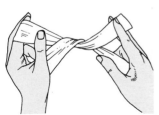

1 Hold one end of the bandage in each hand. Take the left end over the right, and under.

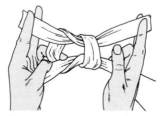

2 Bring the ends up again. Take the right end over the left and under. Pull the knot firm and carefully tuck the ends in.

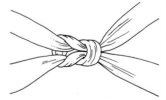

The completed reef knot

SLINGS

These are used to provide support and protection for injured arms, wrists and hands or for immobilizing an upper limb when there are chest injuries. There are two types, the *Arm* sling and the *Elevation* sling. Apply slings from the injured side so that you can provide extra support and protection.

ARM SLING

This sling is used where there are injuries to the upper limb and for some chest injuries. It holds the forearm across the chest but it is effective only if the casualty sits or stands.

When an arm sling is in the correct position, the casualty's hand will be slightly higher than the elbow. The base of the bandage should lie at the root of the little finger, leaving all fingernails exposed.

METHOD

1 Ask the casualty to sit down, and support her forearm on the injured side with her wrist and hand a little higher than her elbow – the casualty may be able to support her own arm.

2 Using the hollow between her elbow and chest, slide one end of the triangular bandage between her chest and forearm so that its point reaches well beyond her elbow.

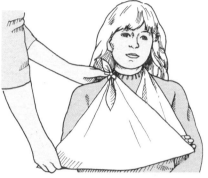

4 Still supporting her forearm, carry the lower end of the bandage up over her forearm and hand, leaving only the fingertips exposed. Using a reef knot, tie on the injured side in the hollow above her collar-bone.

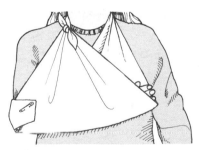

5 Finally, bring the point forward and secure it to the front of the bandage with a safety pin. If no safety pin is available, twist the fold at the point and tuck it between the bandage and the front of the arm.

6 Check the circulation in the limb (see p.175). If it is affected, adjust the bandage and/or position of the sling.

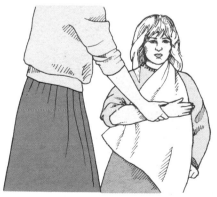

3 Place the upper end over her shoulder on the sound side and around the back of her neck to the front of the injured side.

ELEVATION SLING

This sling is used to support the hand and forearm in a well-raised position if the hand is bleeding, if there are complicated chest injuries or if there are shoulder injuries.

METHOD

1 Ask the casualty to sit down and support his injured limb. Place his forearm across his chest with his fingertips almost resting on his opposite shoulder.

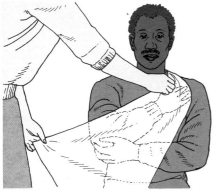

2 Place an open bandage over his forearm and hand with its point reaching well beyond the elbow and its upper end just over the shoulder on the sound side.

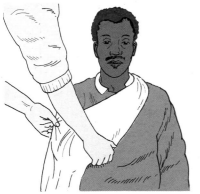

3 Supporting the casualty's forearm, ease the base of the bandage round under his hand, forearm and elbow.

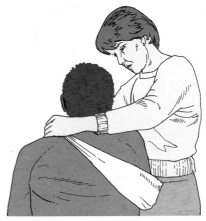

4 Carry the lower end round across his back and over to the front of the uninjured shoulder.

5 Using a reef knot, tie on the sound side in front of the hollow above his collar-bone, gently adjusting the height of the sling if necessary.

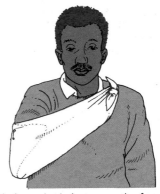

6 Tuck the point in between the forearm and the front part of the bandage. Turn the fold back against the arm and secure it with a safety pin. If a safety pin is not available, tuck the fold over the top of his forearm.

7 Check the circulation in the limb (see p.175). If it is affected, adjust the bandage and/or the position of the sling.

IMPROVISED SLINGS

If no triangular bandages are available, slings may be improvised in several ways to provide adequate support.

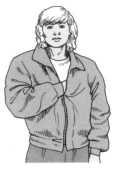 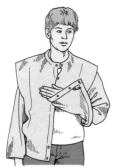 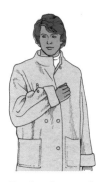 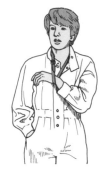

- Support the injured limb in the fastening of a jacket or waistcoat.

- Turn up the lower edge of the casualty's jacket and pin it to her clothing.

- Pin the sleeve of the injured limb to the casualty's clothing.

- Use a scarf, belt, tie or tights to support the injured limb.

HAND/FOOT BANDAGE

This is used for holding a light dressing on to a hand or foot injury such as a graze or burn where pressure is not required. For bandaging a bleeding wound in the palm of the hand, see p.74. Adapt the method below for the feet.

NOTE

For a small hand or foot you may need to fold in a hem along the base of the bandage.

METHOD

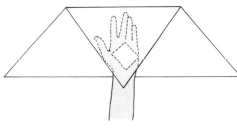 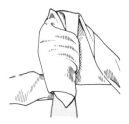 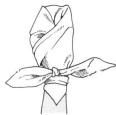

1 Keeping the injury uppermost, place a bandage under the casualty's hand with the base at his or her wrist and the point away from the casualty. Bring the point up over the hand to the wrist.

2 Carry the ends around the hand, cross them and tie off over the wrist below the point, using a reef knot.

3 Bring the point down over the knot and secure (see p.183).

4 Check the circulation (see p.175).

SCALP BANDAGE

This is used to hold a dressing in place over a scalp wound but it is *not* used to control bleeding.

METHOD

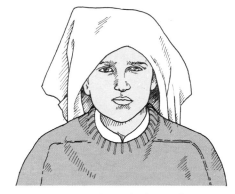

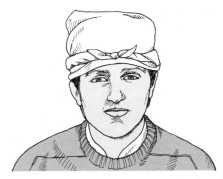

4 Using a reef knot, tie off on his forehead close to the hem.

1 Fold in a hem along the base of a triangular bandage. Place the base on the casualty's forehead so that the centre of the base is above, but close to, his eyebrows and the point of the bandage hangs down at the back of his head.

2 Carry the ends round to the back of his head passing them just above his ears.

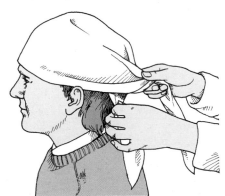

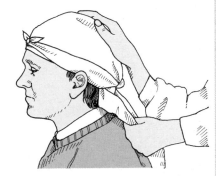

5 Steady his head with one hand and with your other hand, gently draw the point of the bandage down to take up the slack.

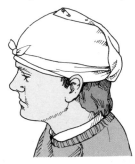

3 Cross the ends above the point of the bandage in the nape of his neck and bring them around to the front.

6 Turn up the point, and secure with a safety pin to the bandage on top of the casualty's head.

ROLLER BANDAGES

This type of bandage can be used to keep dressings in position, to apply pressure to control bleeding or to support a sprain (see p. 133) or a strain (see p. 130). Standard roller bandages are made of cotton, gauze or linen and are usually supplied in 5 m (5 yd) rolls. Crepe and "conforming" bandages hold dressings lightly but firmly in place and, because they mould to the shape of the limb, they maintain an even pressure.

Roller bandages are available in many different sizes. The size and type used will vary according to the part of the body to be bandaged and the size of the casualty (see chart below for details of sizes).

Before applying a roller bandage make sure it is tightly rolled and of a suitable width. Position yourself in front of the injury and support the injured part by hand in the position in which it is to remain. Hold the bandage with the "head" uppermost and unroll only a few centimetres of the bandage at a time. To bandage a left limb hold the bandage in your right hand. To bandage a right limb hold it in your left hand. Always work from the inner side outwards, and from below the injury upwards.

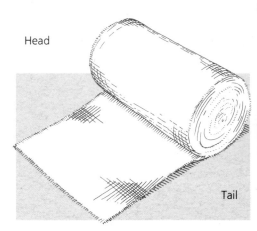

Head

Tail

Parts of a roller bandage
When partly unrolled, the roll of the bandage is called the head and the unrolled part the free end, or tail.

Average sizes of roller bandages for use on an adult

Part to be bandaged	Width
FINGER	2.5 cm (1 in)
HAND	5 cm (2 in)
ARM	5 or 6 cm (2 or 2½ in)
LEG	7.5 or 9 cm (3 or 3½ in)
TRUNK	10 or 15 cm (4 or 6 in)

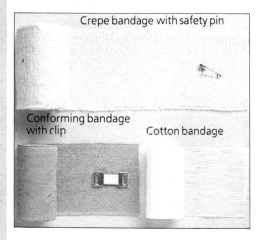

Crepe bandage with safety pin

Conforming bandage with clip

Cotton bandage

APPLYING A ROLLER BANDAGE

The most common method of applying a roller bandage is to use simple spiral turns as shown below. It is used when the part to be bandaged is of uniform width, e.g., forearm.

METHOD

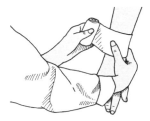

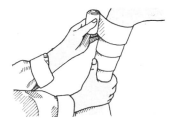

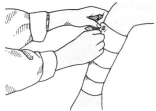

1 Place the tail of the bandage on the limb below the injury and make a firm oblique turn from the inside of the limb outwards to hold the bandage in position.

2 Make a series of spiral turns working up the limb. Allow each successive turn to cover two-thirds of the previous layer and leave the free edges parallel.

3 Finish off with a straight turn and secure the end (see below).

4 Check the circulation (see p.175).

SECURING A ROLLER BANDAGE

1 Finish off above the dressing. Fold in the end of the bandage.

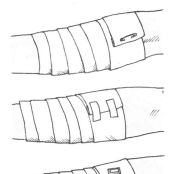

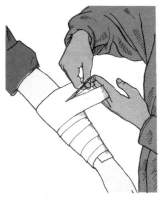

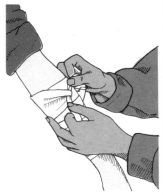

2 Secure with a safety pin, adhesive tape or a bandage clip.

IF pins, tape or clips are not available, gauze bandages can be tied. Leave about 15 cm (6 in) or more of the bandage free – the amount you leave will depend on the size of the part being bandaged – and split it down the centre. Tie a knot at the bottom of the split and, using a reef knot, tie the ends around the limb.

ELBOW/KNEE BANDAGE

The method for bandaging an elbow (shown below) can be adapted for bandaging a knee.

METHOD

1 Ask the casualty to support his limb in the most comfortable position. Place the tail of the bandage on the inside of his elbow and make one straight turn, carrying the head over the elbow tip and around his limb.

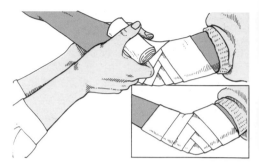

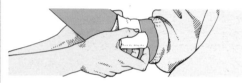

2 Take the bandage around his upper arm, covering half of the first turn, then around his forearm, covering the outer edge of the first turn and touching the edge of the second turn.

3 Continue turns alternately above and below the first turn, allowing each to cover a little more than two-thirds of the previous turn.

4 Finish off with one or two spiral turns above the elbow and secure the end.

5 Check the circulation (see p.175).

HAND/FOOT BANDAGE

To bandage a foot adapt the method for bandaging a hand shown below.

METHOD

1 Ask the casualty to support his hand with his palm held downwards. Fix the tail of the bandage at his wrist by making one straight turn.

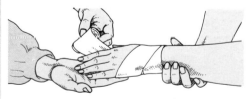

2 Carry the head of the bandage diagonally across the back of his hand towards the base of the little finger, then take it around the palm of the hand under the fingers to the base of the fingernails.

3 Carry the head of the bandage up across the top of the fingers to the root of the nail of the little finger. Then, bring it down around the palm again and diagonally across the back of the hand towards the wrist.

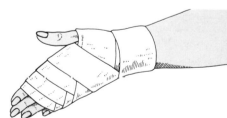

4 Continue making these figure-of-eight turns until the hand is covered. Finish off by making a spiral turn at the wrist and secure the end.

5 Check the circulation (see p.175).

TUBULAR GAUZE BANDAGES

Made of a roll of seamless gauze, these bandages are in many ways easier and quicker to apply than traditional bandages. They are, however, more expensive and require a special applicator.

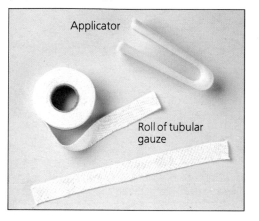

Applicator

Roll of tubular gauze

METHOD

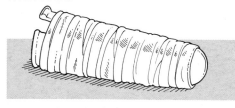

1 Cut a length of the tubular gauze approximately two and a half times the length of the area to be covered. Then push the whole length of the gauze on to the applicator.

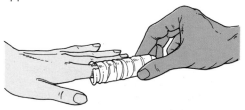

2 Gently push the applicator over the dressing on the finger.

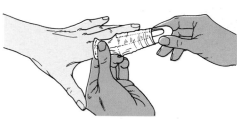

3 Holding the end of the gauze in position with one hand, gently pull back the applicator with your other hand, leaving one length of tubular gauze in position on the limb and the other on the applicator.

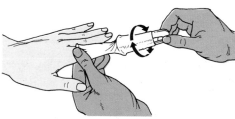

4 Holding the end of the gauze on the limb, twist once or twice, and push it back on to the limb again.

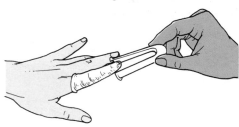

5 Withdraw the applicator leaving two layers of the gauze on the finger.

DO NOT twist the gauze more than twice as you may impede the circulation.

6 Secure the end of the gauze with adhesive strapping.

SPLINTS

These are used to hold fractured or injured limbs, and sometimes the whole body, steady while a casualty is being removed to hospital. Ideally a sound leg can be used to support an injured one by tying bandages around both limbs. This is called "body-splinting". However, if this is not possible, or greater support is required, then a splint will be needed.

The basic requirement of any splint is that it is long enough to extend well beyond the joints above and below the injury and that it is well-padded. When placed against a limb, extra padding should be inserted where the bones are prominent (e.g., at the ankles) and in the natural hollows (e.g., between the legs). For information on when and how to use splints, see *Fractures*, pp. 106–123.

There are many different types of splints available commercially, including inflatable, foam plastic, wood and wire-cage splints. Splints, however, can be improvised by using any material which is rigid, and long and broad enough to support the injured limb. Examples of this are boards, fencing pieces, sticks, brooms and rolled-up newspapers.

Inflatable splints
These are usually made of two concentric tubes of strong transparent plastic, joined together at the ends. They are made in various sizes and are shaped to the upper and lower limbs, and are secured by a zip or Velcro. They are inflated by blowing into an air valve on the outside wall of the outer tube.

Once the splint is blown up, the air pressure inside it will increase as the temperature rises. This helps to comfort and support the injured limb. At the correct pressure, the splint can be indented by firm pressure of the thumb. In this way a conscious patient can monitor the pressure. As well as comforting and supporting a broken limb, inflatable splints have several other advantages: they are easily fitted; they control swelling and bleeding; the limb can be seen and kept under observation; and X-rays can be taken without removing the splint.

Inflatable splints should not be used for thigh or upper arm fractures as the joints above the fracture cannot be immobilized. In addition, they must not be used when the circulation of a limb is likely to be affected, e.g., at the wrist, ankle or elbow.

METHOD OF APPLICATION

1 Empty the appropriate pockets.

2 Whilst holding the fractured limb steady with two hands and applying traction (see p. 109), ask a bystander to slide the opened splint evenly under the limb, to extend well beyond the joints above and below the suspected fracture. The splint may be applied over clothing provided the ridges have been smoothed out.

3 Ask the bystander to secure the zip. Inflate as above.

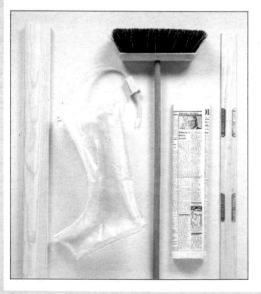

Suitable splints
These include from left to right: a plank, an inflatable splint, a broom, a newspaper and an adjustable splint.

FIRST AID KITS

While bandages and dressings can be improvised, it is far better to have proper equipment on hand. These materials should always be kept in a clean, dry, air-tight container. Do not keep the container in a damp atmosphere, as in a bathroom, and make sure that it is clearly labelled.

The suggested list of contents for a first aid kit (right) should be taken as a guide to the minimum you should have in a kit, although you may add to the list if you wish. For example, it may be considered advisable to keep extra triangular bandages and several 25 g (1 oz) packs of cotton wool. Tweezers and scissors may also be useful.

A first aid kit should include
- 10 individually wrapped sterile adhesive dressings
- 1 sterile eye pad
- 1 triangular bandage
- 1 sterile covering for a serious wound
- 6 safety pins
- 3 medium-sized sterile dressings
- 1 large sterile dressing
- 1 extra large sterile dressing

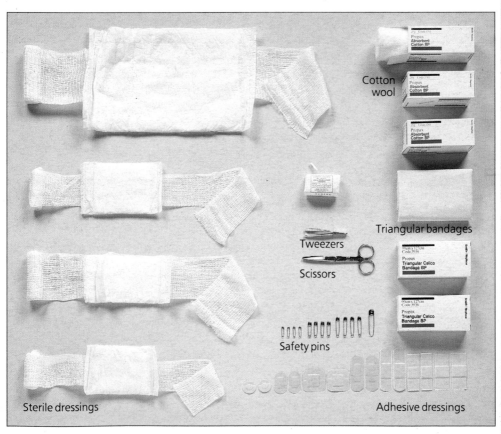

Cotton wool

Triangular bandages

Tweezers

Scissors

Safety pins

Sterile dressings

Adhesive dressings

HANDLING & TRANSPORT

The comfort, safety and well-being of the casualty are among your primary considerations and you must always make sure that the condition will not be made worse by careless handling or movement. The most important rule to remember is: *never move a severely injured or ill person unless there is immediate danger to life or if skilled help is not readily available.* It is better to leave the casualty undisturbed, send for help and provide First Aid on the spot.

If the casualty's life is endangered by fire, falling debris or poisonous gases, move the casualty as quickly as possible without endangering yourself. Otherwise it is important, particularly if the casualty is unconscious, to carry out a quick examination before attempting to move the casualty (see pp.33–37).

There are various methods of carrying casualties using support from one or more helpers. The method used depends on: the nature and severity of the injury; the number of helpers and the facilities available; the casualty's build; the distance to shelter; and the route to be travelled.

Warning *Never move a seriously injured casualty on your own if help is available.* Always make sure that everyone involved, including the casualty, if conscious, knows exactly what is going to happen and what they must do before you begin, and always give a preparatory command before each stage.

If the casualty is to be removed to hospital, arrange for an ambulance, although, if the injuries are minor or only involve the upper limb, the casualty can be taken in a car. Whichever method of transport is used, the aim is always the same – to enable the casualty to reach hospital without deterioration or discomfort. Wherever possible, the position in which the casualty is found or has been placed should not be changed and the general condition watched carefully throughout.

LIFTING CASUALTIES

This is a skill and, if it is done correctly, even a very heavy casualty can be lifted without undue strain. However, it is important that you should not attempt to lift too heavy a weight and that you always obtain assistance from any available bystanders in order to avoid injury to yourself.

There are two principles of lifting: first, you should always use the most powerful muscles – those of the thigh, hip and shoulder; second, the weight should be kept as close to your body as possible.

It is very important that the correct posture for lifting is adopted. Feet should be placed comfortably apart to ensure a stable, balanced posture and a firm stance. Keep your back straight and head erect and hold the casualty close to your body using your shoulders to support the weight. Use your whole hand to strengthen the grasp. If the casualty begins to slip, do not injure your own back by trying to prevent him or her falling. Let the casualty slide slowly and gently to the ground without causing more damage to the injured area.

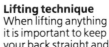

Lifting technique
When lifting anything it is important to keep your back straight and bend at the knees if necessary.

CARRIES FOR ONE FIRST AIDER

If help is available, *do not* attempt to move a seriously ill or injured casualty on your own.

CRADLE METHOD
To carry lightweight casualties or children, pass one arm under the casualty's thighs and the other around the trunk above the waist and lift.

DRAG METHOD
This method involves pulling the casualty along the ground without lifting. It should *only* be used where a casualty is unable to stand and must be moved quickly from a source of danger.

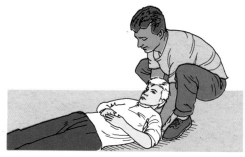

1 Fold the casualty's arms across her chest and crouch behind her head. Place your hands under her shoulders, grasp her armpits and cradle her head on your forearms.

2 Pull her along the ground.

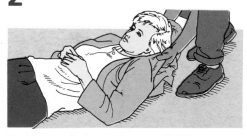

IF the casualty is wearing a jacket or coat, unbutton it and pull it back up under her head. Pull her along the ground in the same way with her head supported on the coat.

HUMAN CRUTCH
This is used to support a conscious casualty who is able to walk with assistance. It should *not* be used if an upper limb is injured.

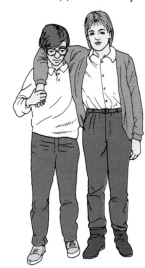

1 Stand at the casualty's injured side, if any. Place his nearest arm around your neck and hold his hand with your free hand.

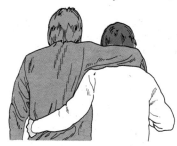

2 Put your other arm around his waist and grasp his clothing. The casualty may be given additional support from a walking stick or staff.

PICK-A-BACK
If the casualty is small, light, conscious and able to hold on to you, carry him in the "pick-a-back" fashion.

FIREMAN'S LIFT

This method is used to move a conscious or unconscious child or a lightweight adult when you need to keep a hand free.

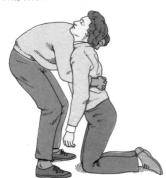
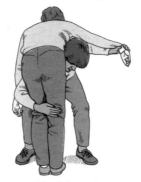
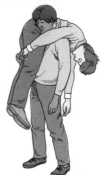

1 Help the casualty to stand up. If he is unconscious or unable to stand, turn him face-down and stand at his head. Place your arms under his armpits and raise him on to his knees and then his feet.

2 Grasp his right wrist with your left hand. Bend down with your head under his extended right arm so that your shoulder is level with his lower abdomen; allow him to fall gently across your shoulders. Place your right arm between or around his legs.

3 Taking the weight on your right shoulder, stand up and gently pull him across both shoulders. Transfer his right wrist to your right hand, leaving your left hand free.

CARRIES FOR TWO FIRST AIDERS

There is a variety of lifts suitable for transporting a casualty with two First Aiders.

FOUR-HANDED SEAT

This method is used to carry a conscious casualty who can assist the bearers by using one or both arms to hold on.

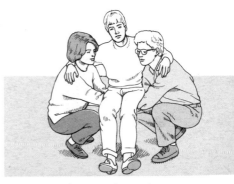

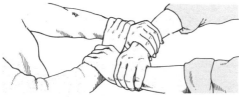

1 Stand facing each other behind the casualty. Make a seat by grasping your own left wrists with your right hands and your partner's right wrist with the free hand; then squat down beside the casualty.

2 Instruct the casualty to place an arm around each of you at the neck, to sit back on to your hands and to steady himself during transport.

3 Rise together, step off with your outside feet and walk with cross-over steps.

TWO-HANDED SEAT

This method is used to carry a casualty who is unable to assist the bearers.

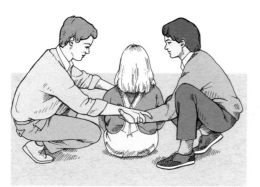

1 Squat facing each other on either side of the casualty. Pass your arms nearest the casualty's body under and around her back just below her shoulders and, if possible, grasp each other's forearms or the casualty's clothing at the waist.

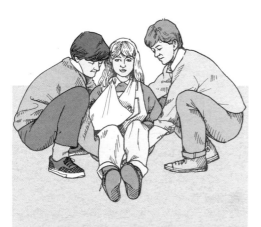

2 Raise the casualty's legs slightly, pass your other arms under the middle of her thighs and grasp each other's wrists.

3 Rise together, step off with your outside feet and walk with cross-over steps.

FORE-&-AFT CARRY

This method can be used to place the casualty on a chair or a carrying chair.

1 Supporting the casualty on both sides, both First Aiders should help the casualty to sit up and fold her arms across her chest.

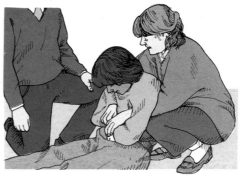

2 One person should move around behind her and place the arms through and under her armpits and grasp her forearms.

DO NOT use this method if the upper limb is injured.

3 The other bearer should remain at her side and place one arm around her back and the other under her thighs.

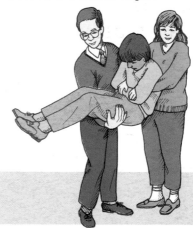

4 Working together, lift the casualty on to the chair or stretcher.

CHAIR METHOD

When a conscious casualty with no serious injuries is to be moved up or down stairs or along passageways, the casualty can be seated on an ordinary chair and carried by two people. However, the passages must be cleared of any obstructions or dangers such as loose matting before you start.

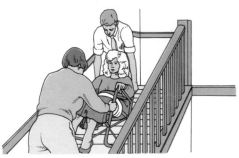

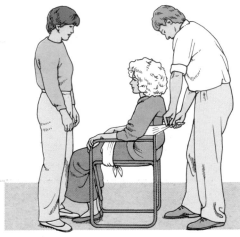

1 Test the chair to ensure that it is strong enough to support the casualty, then sit her down and secure her in position with broad bandages. Stand facing each other, one in front of the chair and one behind.

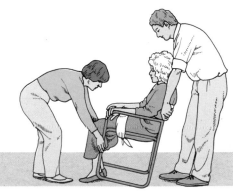

2 The person behind the chair should support the back of the chair and the casualty; the other should hold the chair by the front legs. Slowly tilt the chair backwards to seat the casualty securely then lift together.

3 With the casualty facing forwards, move slowly along the passage or stairs.

IF space permits, you can both stand facing the side of the chair, each supporting the back and the top of a front leg.

LIFTING A CASUALTY IN A WHEELCHAIR

Wheelchair-bound casualties can be transported where they sit by adapting the chair method.

1 Locate the brakes (ask the casualty) and apply securely.

2 Sit the casualty well back in the chair.

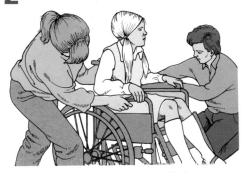

3 Examine the wheelchair to find out which parts are fixed – arm rests and side supports are often removable and will detach if you use them to lift the chair. Supporting the chair from either side, lift by holding the fixed parts, *never* by the wheels.

4 Carry the chair as described above.

STRETCHERS

These are used to carry a seriously ill or injured casualty to an ambulance or similar shelter to minimize the risk of further injury. The stretchers in general use include: the standard stretcher; the scoop stretcher; the trolley bed; the Utila folding stretcher; the pole-and-canvas stretcher; the carrying sheet; the carrying chair; the Neil Robertson stretcher; and the paraguard stretcher.

Most stretchers can be used to transport casualties with any injury and should be rigid enough to carry casualties with a suspected spine fracture without additional boards. All equipment must be tested *before* it is used.

Testing a stretcher
To ensure that a stretcher is capable of taking the weight of a casualty, one person should lie on the stretcher and each end of the stretcher should be lifted in turn. Then, both ends should be lifted at the same time.

> ### NOTE
> If possible, test the stretcher before leaving an ambulance station and not in front of a casualty.

THE STANDARD STRETCHER

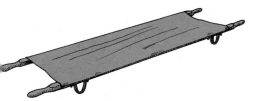

The "standard" or Furley stretcher consists of poles, handles, traverses, runners and a canvas bed. The traverses are jointed so that the stretcher can be opened and closed. When closed, the poles lie close together with the canvas bed folded on top. This is then kept in position by two transverse straps. If slings are carried they are laid along the canvas held by the straps.

Opening the stretcher
1 Place the stretcher on its side with its runners towards you and the studs or buckles securing the straps uppermost. Unfasten any straps.

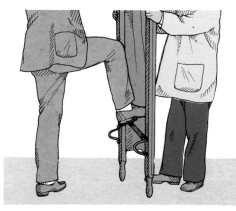

2 Push the traverses fully open with your foot, whilst placing the stretcher upright on either end.

Closing the stretcher
1 Turn the stretcher on its side with its runners towards you and the studs or buckles which secure the straps uppermost. Push the joints of the traverses inwards with your heel to release them.

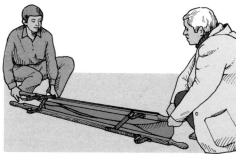

2 Push the poles together, pulling the canvas out from between them. Fold the canvas neatly on to the poles and secure with the straps.

SCOOP STRETCHER

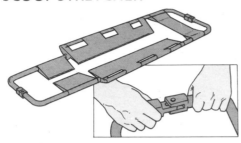

The scoop, or orthopaedic, stretcher is an adjustable stretcher used to lift casualties on to an ambulance trolley bed without altering the position in which they were found. It is not used to carry a casualty any distance. The length can be adjusted to suit any size of casualty and because he or she does not have to be moved, it is particularly useful for picking up a casualty with a suspected spinal fracture (see pp.96 and 125) or internal injuries. Remove hard objects from the casualty's pocket.

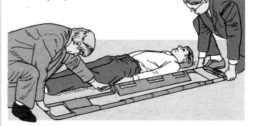

1 Bring the stretcher to the casualty's side and adjust the length.

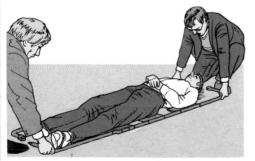

2 Uncouple both ends of the stretcher and gently slip each half of the stretcher under the casualty; rejoin the head sections.

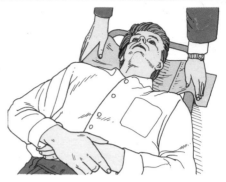

3 Place the head pad in position.

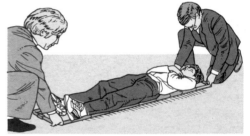

4 While one First Aider stays at the head, the other should rejoin the foot section. Secure the head pad to the stretcher.

5 Working from either side of the stretcher, lift it and the casualty and place on the trolley bed. Uncouple the stretcher and remove it.

TROLLEY BED

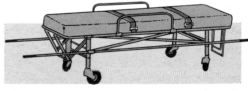

This fully-adjustable stretcher bed on wheels is made of light metal and is carried in many ambulances.

Trolley beds should always be kept prepared for immediate use. A canvas sheet from a pole-and-canvas stretcher is laid on the stretcher bed and two blankets are placed on top (see p.197).

UTILA FOLDING STRETCHER

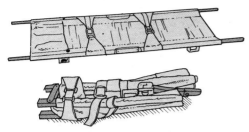

This is a lightweight version of the standard stretcher. It has light metal poles with telescopic handles and a canvas or plastic bed. The folding stretcher is available in two versions: one folds in the same way as the standard stretcher; the other folds in half in the centre and so takes up less space.

POLE-&-CANVAS STRETCHER

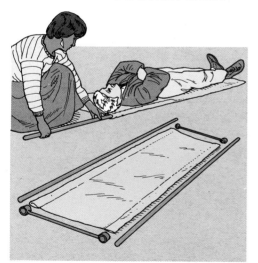

This is one of the most commonly used stretchers. It consists of a canvas or plastic sheet about 200 cm (80 in) long and 50 cm (20 in) wide and two long poles. The canvas can be folded and slid under the casualty where he or she lies (see p.198). The poles are passed through sleeves down the side of the canvas to form the stretcher. Spacer bars may be placed over the ends of the poles to keep them apart and the stretcher firm.

NEIL ROBERTSON STRETCHER

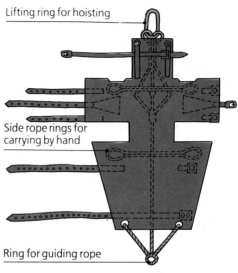

Lifting ring for hoisting

Side rope rings for carrying by hand

Ring for guiding rope

Made of stout canvas and bamboo, this stretcher is designed for lifting casualties in the *upright* position through small hatches, e.g., manholes or pot-hole entrances, or for lowering casualties from heights, as in mountain rescue.

The casualty is placed on the stretcher. The strap at the top is passed around the casualty's forehead to hold his or her head in position. The upper flaps are wrapped around the chest and secured with the two short straps, leaving the arms outside. These are then secured with the long strap. However, if the casualty is unconscious, his or her arms are left inside the canvas. The lower flaps are strapped round the lower limbs.

The ring at the head of the stretcher is used for hoisting. The side rope rings should be used only for carrying by hand, and should *never* be used as an aid to hoist the casualty by ropes or lines. Another length of rope is attached to the ring at the foot of the stretcher to guide it.

The stretcher should be stored in a place where it is most likely to be needed together with a suitable length of rope, preferably made of a rot-proof fibre.

PARAGUARD STRETCHER

This stretcher is similar to the Neil Robertson stretcher and is used for the same purposes. However, it is lighter, less cumbersome and more durable than the Neil Robertson and can be folded up and carried on the back. The main advantage of the paraguard stretcher is that it will bend in the middle so you can negotiate obstacles.

IMPROVISED STRETCHERS

> **NOTE**
> Always test an improvised stretcher (see *Testing a stretcher*, p.193).

Stretchers may be improvised as follows:
■ Tie broad-fold bandages at intervals around two strong poles.
■ Spread out a rug, piece of sacking, tarpaulin or a strong blanket and roll up two strong poles in the sides.

■ Use a hurdle, broad piece of wood, door or shutter and add a rug, clothing, or straw covered with a piece of stout cloth or sacking.

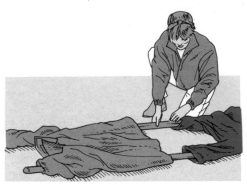

■ Turn the sleeves of two or three coats inside out. Pass two strong poles through the sleeves and button up the coats. The poles may be kept apart by strips of wood tied to the poles at each end of the stretcher.

PREPARING A STRETCHER OR TROLLEY BED

To protect and keep the casualty warm, blanket the stretcher according to the number of blankets available.

WITH ONE BLANKET

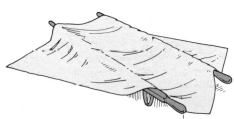

1 Place the blanket diagonally over the stretcher so that there are two opposing corners at the ends of the stretcher.

2 After placing the casualty on the stretcher, bring the point of the blanket at the foot of the stretcher up over his feet and tuck a small fold between his ankles.

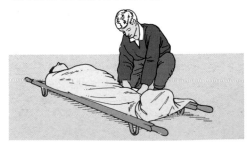

3 Bring the lower side of the blanket over his legs and tuck it in. Fold the point of the blanket at the head around his head and neck. Then bring the upper side of the blanket over his trunk and tuck it in.

WITH TWO BLANKETS

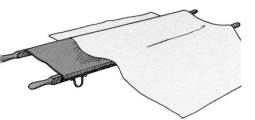

1 Place the first blanket lengthwise across the stretcher with one edge covering half the handles at the head and leaving slightly more material to one side of the stretcher than the other.

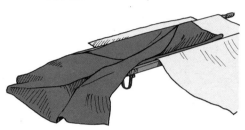

2 Fold the second blanket lengthwise into three and place on the stretcher with the upper edge about one third of the way down the stretcher, leaving enough at the bottom end to fold in over the feet.

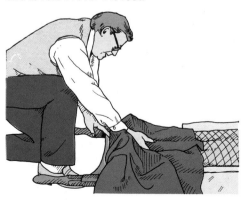

3 After placing the casualty on the stretcher, open the foot of the top blanket and bring it up over her feet and tuck a small fold between her ankles to prevent them rubbing.

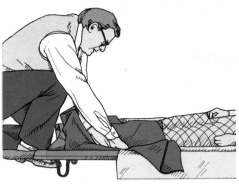

4 Bring the folds of the blanket over her legs and feet and tuck them in.

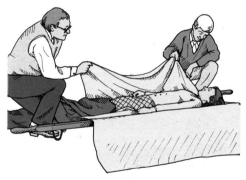

5 Turn in the upper corners of the first blanket and bring the shorter side over the casualty and tuck it in.

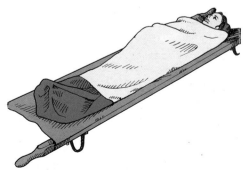

6 Finally, bring the long side of the blanket over the casualty and tuck it in.

LOADING A STRETCHER

Ideally, five people will be required to load a casualty on to a stretcher – four to lift the casualty and one to move the stretcher. However, there are methods of moving a casualty using two or three bearers if there are not enough people available or space is limited. The First Aider in charge of the casualty should assemble a squad of four bearers, decide which method of lifting is to be used, make it clear to each person what is to be done and give *all* the directions.

If you are unloading a stretcher in order to place a casualty on to a bed or examination couch, reverse the loading procedure.

LOADING A CASUALTY ON TO A POLE-&-CANVAS STRETCHER

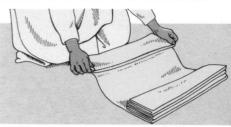

1 Working from top and bottom, fold the canvas sheet into a concertina shape; make three complete folds from the top and four from the bottom. Slide the folded canvas under the casualty through the hollow of his back. Alternatively, adopt the procedure for a blanket lift (see p.200).

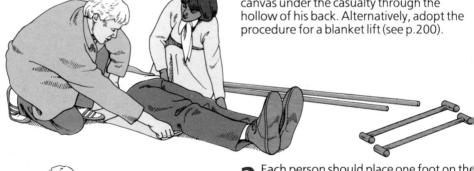

2 Each person should place one foot on the top pile of folds, pull the casualty's clothing taut from his waist down and gently work the canvas down under his buttocks and legs. Repeat for the top part of his body until the canvas is extended.

3 Working from the casualty's head, slide the poles into the sleeves and place spacer bars over the ends if they are to be used. Lift the stretcher as described on pp.203–205.

PLACING A BLANKET UNDER A CASUALTY

> **NOTE**
> This method can also be used to load a pole-and-canvas stretcher.
>   A firmer lift may be achieved by folding the blanket in half lengthwise, and proceeding as from step 2 below.

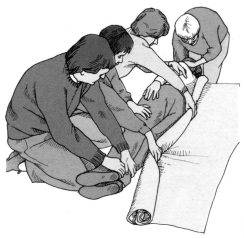

3 All four bearers should kneel at the side of the casualty, opposite to the blanket and turn her slowly and gently on to her side towards them. Move the rolled portion of the blanket or rug up against her back.

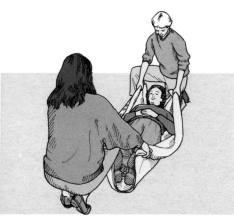

1 To test the blanket or rug, lay it on the ground. One person should lie down on it while two others attempt to lift it. If it is strong enough, proceed with steps 2–4.

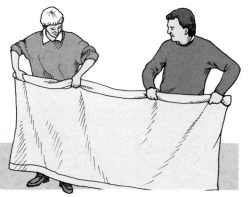

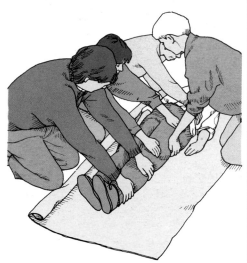

2 Roll the blanket or rug lengthwise for half its width; place the roll in line with and against the injured side of the casualty (or most severely injured side if both are injured).

4 Gently turn the casualty on to her back over the roll of blanket and turn her far enough on to her other side to allow the blanket to be unrolled. Turn her on to her back again.

BLANKET LIFT

1 Stand so that two bearers face each other on either side of the casualty's trunk, and two face each other at his lower limbs. Tightly roll the two edges of the blanket up against his side.

IF poles of sufficient length and rigidity are available, the edges of the blanket can be rolled around them. It will make the casualty easier to lift and prevent the blanket sagging.

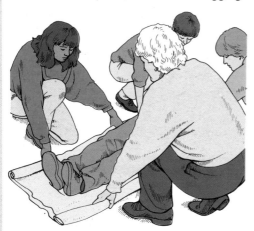

2 With backs straight, squat and grasp the blanket with your palms downwards and fingers at the inner side of the rolled blanket edge. The two bearers nearest the casualty's head should each place one hand level with his head and the other at his waist. The bearers at the lower limbs should place one hand level with his hips and one at his ankles.

3 Working together, lean back and carefully and evenly lift the casualty high enough to enable a fifth person to push a stretcher underneath.

4 Working together, carefully and evenly lower the casualty on to the stretcher.

IF a fifth person is not available or if it is not possible to push the stretcher under the casualty, place the stretcher in line with him as close to his head as possible. Carefully lift him and move with short even side paces until he is directly over the stretcher, then lower him on to it.

MANUAL LIFTS

If a blanket is not available you will have to lift the casualty using one of the following methods.

For four bearers

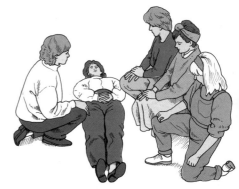

1 Three bearers should place themselves on the left of the casualty: one facing her knees, one facing her hips and the third facing her shoulders. The bearer in charge of the casualty should be on her right facing the middle bearer.

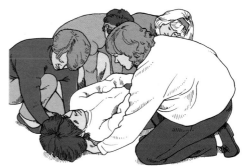

2 All bearers should go down on their left knees and place their forearms beneath the casualty, paying particular attention to the site of the injury. The person in charge should grasp the left wrist of the bearer at the shoulders with his left hand and the right wrist of the bearer opposite with his right hand. The person at the shoulders should support the head and shoulders and ensure an open airway, and the fourth bearer should support the lower limbs.

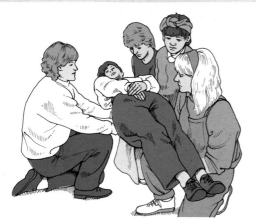

3 When the order "lift" is given by the person in charge, raise the casualty gently, slowly and evenly and place on the knees of the other three bearers.

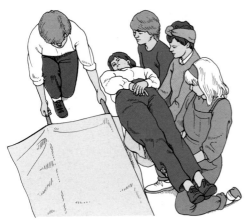

4 If a fifth person is not available to move the stretcher, the person in charge should disengage, get the prepared stretcher and place it under the casualty. It should be positioned so that the casualty's head will be just clear of the top traverse when lowered on to it. The bearer should then resume his original position and rejoin hands.

5 When the order "lower" is given, work together and raise the casualty slightly from the bearer's knees. Then slowly and evenly lower the casualty on to the stretcher or trolley bed.

For three bearers

1 Place the stretcher in line with the casualty as near his head as possible. One bearer should kneel on one knee on the injured side of the casualty level with his knees and place his hands under the casualty's legs. The other two should kneel on opposite sides of the casualty's chest and grasp each other's wrists under the casualty's shoulders and hips.

2 On the order "lift", gently and evenly raise the casualty and stand up. Then, moving with side paces, carry the casualty head first over the stretcher.

3 When the order "lower" is given, gently, slowly and evenly lower the casualty on to the stretcher.

IF the casualty is seriously injured and must be kept rigid, all three bearers should work from the same side. They should raise him and tilt his body towards them as they lift.

LOADING A CASUALTY IN THE RECOVERY POSITION

1 Prepare the stretcher as on p.196 but place one extra rolled blanket down one side of the stretcher to support the casualty in the Recovery Position (see p.24).

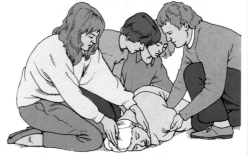

2 Bring the casualty's arms down by her side; three bearers should squat at the back of the casualty, arranged at her head to ensure an open airway, at her hips and at her knees, while a fourth person supports the casualty's trunk from the other side.

3 Follow the procedure described left and above.

MANUAL LIFT FOR A FRACTURED SPINE

If the casualty has a fractured spine, do not move him unless it is unavoidable (see pp.96 and 125). However, there are certain occasions when you may have to lift the casualty on to a stretcher: if there is no scoop or similar stretcher available; if the use of a scoop stretcher is impossible, e.g., on very soft ground; if the ambulance cannot reach the site of the accident; or if danger dictates emergency movement.

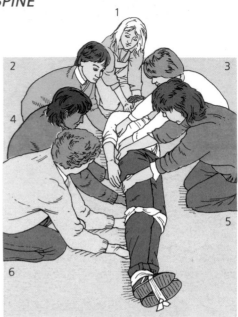

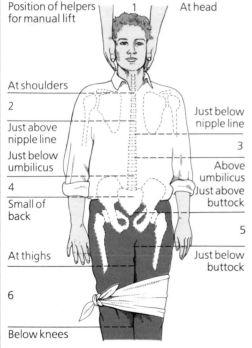

Position of helpers for manual lift

1 — At head

At shoulders
2 — Just below nipple line
3

Just above nipple line
Just below umbilicus — Above umbilicus / Just above buttock
4
Small of back
5 — Just below buttock

At thighs

6

Below knees

1 One person should kneel at the casualty's head and support his head and neck in the normal neutral position (see p.96).

2 Remove hard objects from pockets. Place adequate soft padding between his legs. Tie a figure-of-eight bandage at his feet and ankles, and a broad-fold bandage around his knees. Place his arms across his chest.

3 Five helpers should remove all rings, watches etc., then kneel on their right knees beside the casualty as shown above — three on one side, and two on the other.

4 The team of two should place their arms on the casualty's far side. At the command of the head holder, they should turn the casualty towards them using the log roll method, just high enough to allow the team of three to insert their arms under the casualty as far as their elbows.

5 The team of two should lower the casualty on to the team of three's arms, then insert their arms under the casualty between helpers 2 and 4, and 4 and 6.

DO NOT cross or hold hands.

6 To the head holder's command, gently and evenly lift the casualty high enough to let the stretcher in.

7 A prepared stretcher should be placed under the casualty by other helpers.

8 Working together, gently lower the casualty on to the stretcher so that his head is just clear of the top traverse. Carefully remove your hands.

CARRYING A STRETCHER

When the casualty has been placed on the stretcher, the bearers should take up their positions at each end of the stretcher. At least two trained bearers will be required to carry a stretcher and the person in charge of the casualty should always remain at the casualty's head. If bystanders are available, they should be used to help carry the stretcher to spread the load. However, there should be at least one trained bearer at each end of the stretcher.

Unless a casualty is suffering from shock, the head should be kept higher than the feet So, as a general rule, the casualty should always be carried feet first. However, there are a few exceptions:

■ When going up stairs or hills when the lower limbs are *not* injured.

■ When going down stairs or hills when the casualty's lower limbs *are* injured or the casualty is suffering from hypothermia.
■ When carrying a casualty to the side or foot of a bed.
■ When loading a casualty into an ambulance.

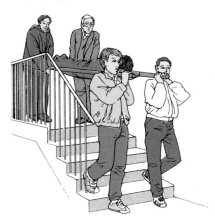

Moving down stairs
Carry the casualty down stairs head first if his lower limbs are injured.

FOR FOUR BEARERS

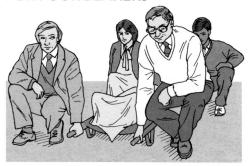

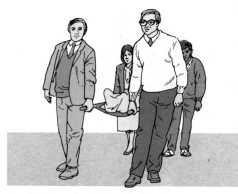

1 Keeping their backs straight, all the bearers should squat and grasp the handles with their inner hands, palms inwards. When the order "lift" is given by the person in charge, all rise together, holding the stretcher with arms fully extended and keeping it level.

2 At the order "advance", move together, stepping off with the foot nearest the stretcher and walking with a short, flat-footed pace to avoid bouncing the stretcher.

3 When you reach the ambulance, working together, gently and evenly lower the stretcher to the ground with the casualty's head nearest the ambulance.

CROSSING UNEVEN GROUND

If possible, four bearers should carry a stretcher when crossing uneven ground. Secure the casualty to the stretcher with a harness or broad-fold bandages before you start. Keep the stretcher as nearly level as possible; this can be done by each bearer adjusting the height of the stretcher individually.

If crossing very uneven ground for a short distance, the four bearers should stand at the side of the stretcher facing inwards. Grasp the poles with one hand and place the other about 75 cm (30 in) in from the end of the stretcher; then, move with side paces and *not* cross-over steps.

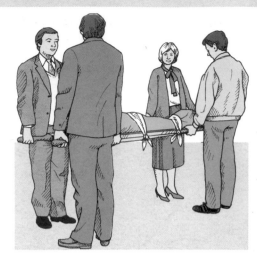

CROSSING A WALL

Always avoid crossing a wall, if possible, even if it means carrying a stretcher further. However, if there is no gap, follow the procedure described below.

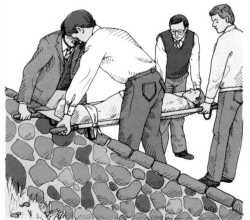

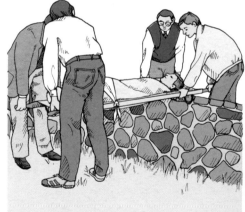

1 Lower the stretcher in front of the wall and turn inwards. Lift the stretcher and rest it on the wall, with the front runners beyond the wall.

2 The front bearers should cross the wall one at a time while the others steady the stretcher.

3 All the bearers should lift the stretcher again and move it forward until the rear runners are close to the approach side of the wall. The remaining bearers then cross the wall one at a time while the others steady the stretcher.

4 Finally, lower the stretcher to the ground then carry it in the usual way.

MOVING A STRETCHER FROM ONE LEVEL TO ANOTHER

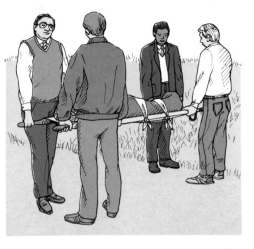 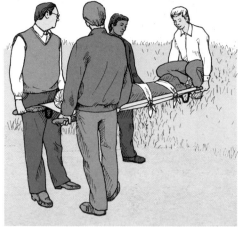

1 All the bearers should stand at the side of the stretcher as shown for crossing uneven ground (see opposite). Lift the stretcher so that it is level with the top of the bank and place the foot of the stretcher on the bank.

2 One bearer should then get up on to the bank ready to receive the stretcher while the others move it forward.

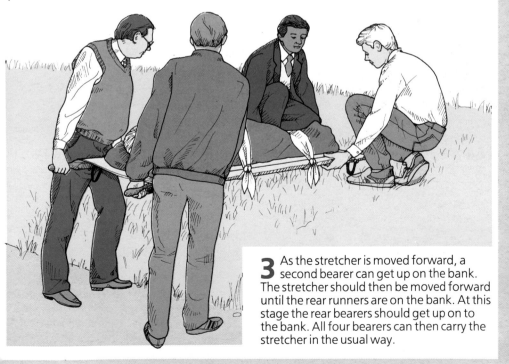

3 As the stretcher is moved forward, a second bearer can get up on the bank. The stretcher should then be moved forward until the rear runners are on the bank. At this stage the rear bearers should get up on to the bank. All four bearers can then carry the stretcher in the usual way.

LOADING AN AMBULANCE

A few ambulances have flat built-in beds with grooves to take the runners of a standard stretcher. Four people will be required to load this ambulance: one to stand inside the ambulance ready to guide the stretcher, while the other three stand one on either side of the stretcher and one at the end ready to lift. If there are two berths, always load the left one first.

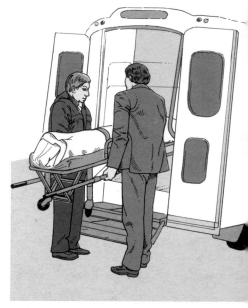

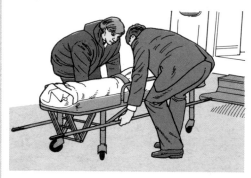

1 If loading a trolley bed into an ambulance, two bearers should take up their positions one at each side of the trolley bed.

2 Working together, raise the trolley bed to the required height and feed/push it head first into the ambulance.

UNLOADING AN AMBULANCE

One bearer takes hold of the handles at the rear while another bearer holds the handles at the head in the ambulance. The bearer at the rear gently withdraws the stretcher or trolley bed. As it is withdrawn, two bearers, one on each side of the trolley bed, support it, moving with side paces until the end is clear of the ambulance. The bearer in the ambulance then gets down, takes the handles at the head and helps to lower the trolley bed or stretcher to the ground.

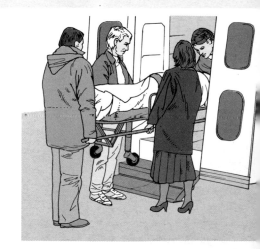

EMERGENCY CHILDBIRTH

There are two situations where you may need to administer First Aid to a pregnant woman: miscarriage or childbirth. In both cases you should seek expert help as soon as possible and be prepared to respond if it should become necessary.

MISCARRIAGE

A miscarriage or "spontaneous abortion" is the loss of the embryo or foetus at any time before the 28th week of pregnancy. It is usually due to abnormality or death of the foetus and is therefore a protective mechanism that avoids the full development and birth of an abnormal baby.

About 20 per cent of all pregnancies end in miscarriage. Although some women may experience a "threatened" miscarriage involving only slight vaginal bleeding, complete miscarriages always include the very real danger of severe vaginal bleeding. Incomplete miscarriage is serious because products of the conception are retained in the womb resulting in severe bleeding.

SYMPTOMS & SIGNS

■ Vaginal bleeding (see p.80) and, if severe, symptoms and signs of shock (see p.86).
■ Cramp-like pains in the lower abdomen or pelvic area; these may be severe.
■ Passage of the foetus and other products of conception.

AIM

Reassure and comfort the casualty and arrange urgent removal to hospital.

TREATMENT

1 Reassure the casualty and keep her warm. Lay her down with her head and shoulders raised and knees slighly bent, supported by a cushion or blanket.

2 Check her pulse (see p.85) and breathing rate (see p.12).

3 Place a sanitary pad or clean towel over her vagina.

4 Keep any material products of conception for medical inspection.

5 If bleeding is continuous and severe, minimize shock by treating as on p.86. If the woman is lying on a bed, raise the foot 30–45 cm (12–18 in).

6 Arrange urgent removal to hospital.

CHILDBIRTH

A woman may go into labour unexpectedly at a time and place where she is unable to put her arrangements for confinement into practice. Also, a few women make no preparation at all.

It is important to remember that childbirth is a natural process and that the majority of births do not threaten the life of either mother or baby. In most cases, there is time to arrange transport to hospital, or for the assistance of a doctor or midwife, but it is nonetheless essential that you clearly understand what you can do and what you should not do, before expert help arrives.

In a normal birth, the baby's head will emerge first. Rarely, however, the baby's position in the womb is reversed and it emerges bottom (breech) first. This requires urgent medical attention.

Never try to delay a birth in any way. Allow the delivery to proceed without interfering until the baby's head is emerging.

THE STAGES OF CHILDBIRTH

Labour is divided into three stages:
- First stage – dilation of the cervix.
- Second stage – delivery of the baby.
- Third stage – delivery of the afterbirth (placenta).

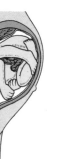
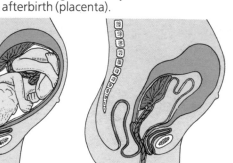

Early first stage | Early second stage | Third stage

THE FIRST STAGE

The first indication that labour has started is when the mother notices cramp-like pains in her abdomen or a low backache. A "show" of blood-stained mucus may be a sign that the neck of the womb (cervix) has begun to dilate and the mucus plug has come away. At this stage the womb (uterus) contracts every 10–20 minutes, dilating the neck of the womb.

This stage may take 12–14 hours for a first child but less for any subsequent pregnancy.

Towards the end of the first stage, the cramp-like contractions become more prolonged, stronger and more frequent. The "waters" will break, indicating that the membranous bag containing the amniotic fluid in which the baby lies has ruptured. The liquid may escape in a sudden rush, although sometimes a constant trickle is all that is evident. When this occurs, it means that the second stage of labour has begun, the baby is on its way and the mother needs help. Preparation for emergency delivery should be made.

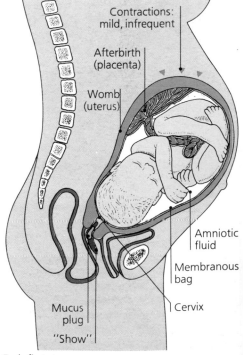

Contractions: mild, infrequent

Afterbirth (placenta)

Womb (uterus)

Amniotic fluid

Membranous bag

Cervix

Mucus plug

"Show"

Early first stage

PREPARING FOR THE BIRTH

The prospective mother is likely to be nervous and excited. Keep calm and reassure her. Arrange a warm, quiet environment and invite assistance from a female relative or neighbour. The father may wish to be present.

Protect the bed, sofa or floor with plastic sheeting, towels or newspaper. If the mother is not at home or near a bed, she can adopt a semi-recumbent position on the floor, the seat of a car, or any flat surface. In a public place, ask any bystanders to stand with their backs to her to screen her from view.

Lay the mother in a semi-recumbent position with her knees drawn up and her head and shoulders comfortably supported. Ask her to remove any clothing that will interfere with the delivery. Put cotton, lint or any suitable sheeting under her buttocks for warmth, and to absorb any subsequent

mess. Cover her with blankets for as long as is possible. Fold a blanket in three and wrap it in a sheet to make a pack to cover the top half of her body during the delivery.

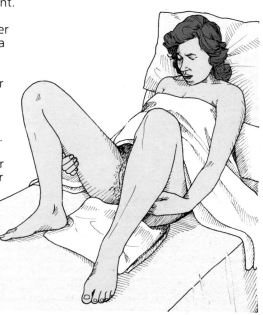

FOR THE BABY

Make sure there is some form of heating available if possible. Prepare a cot, improvised from a basket, drawers or box, and have a blanket, shawl or towel ready to wrap up the baby.

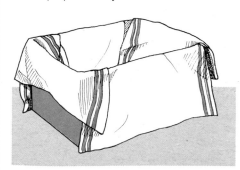

FOR THE DELIVERY

Fill some jugs with hot water and find a clean basin, and a plastic or stout paper bag to hold the soiled swabs, etc. Prepare blunt pointed scissors and three pieces of string 25 cm (9 in) long in case you need to cut the umbilical cord. Boil the scissors and string for 10 minutes or soak in methylated spirits for 10 minutes. Sterile dressings (see p. 171) will be required to dress the cord after cutting.

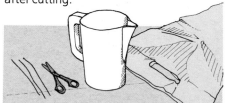

PREVENTING INFECTION

Lack of scrupulous cleanliness can jeopardize the lives of both the mother and the baby. No person who has a cold, sore throat or septic hands should help with the delivery. You and your assistant should both wear masks. If none are available, you can improvise by tying clean handkerchiefs around your faces. If possible, scrub your hands, nails and forearms thoroughly under running water for four minutes. Do not dry them and if they become soiled, wash them again in the same way. After delivery is complete and your help is no longer required, wash your hands thoroughly.

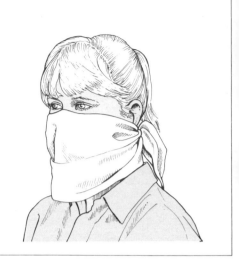

THE SECOND STAGE

It is during this stage that the baby will be born. It generally lasts about one hour for a first baby and may be much shorter for any subsequent births.

Do not move the mother. Remain calm and, if an ambulance has not been summoned, immediately despatch someone to call for one. Instruct him or her to give the ambulance control details of the stage of labour that has been reached, together with the name, if any, of the hospital into which the mother is booked and the address where she can now be found (see *Calling for Assistance*, p.32).

During contractions the mother should be encouraged to grasp her knees, bend her head forward, hold her breath and push downwards, and then to relax between contractions. These will become stronger, prolonged and more frequent (every two to three minutes).

Eventually the perineum (the tissues between the vagina and anus) will become distended, a bulge will appear, and you will see the baby's head at the lower end of the birth canal. This indicates that the baby's birth is imminent.

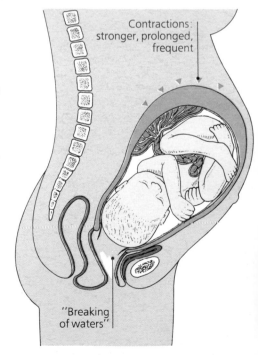

Contractions: stronger, prolonged, frequent

"Breaking of waters"

Early second stage

PROCEDURE FOR DELIVERY

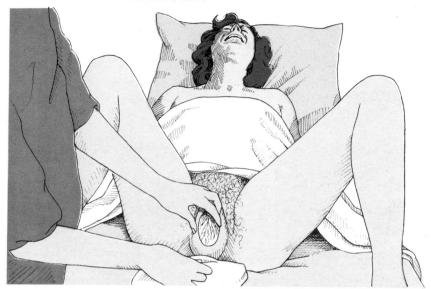

1 Support the head as it begins to appear at the lower end of the birth canal, and hold a clean pad over the back passage (anus). If a bowel movement occurs, wipe it from front to back to avoid soiling the birth canal. During each contraction continue supporting the baby's head until the widest part (crown) of the head is passing through the lower end of the birth canal. Tell the mother to stop pushing, open her mouth and pant.

IF there is a membrane over the baby's face, remove it by tearing it with your fingers. Check at the baby's neck to ensure that the umbilical cord is not around the neck.

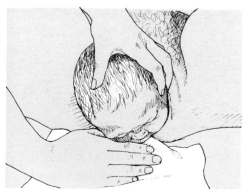

2 Gently support the baby's head as it emerges and steady it to prevent it "shooting" out.

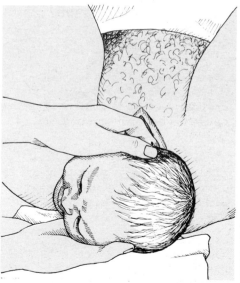

3 The baby's head will rotate and face to the side. Allow this to happen naturally whilst supporting the head.

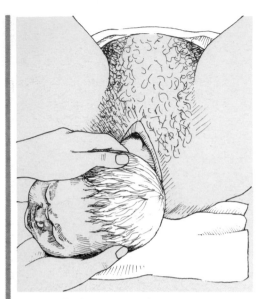

4 Continuing support, lower the baby's head until the uppermost shoulder appears at the birth canal.

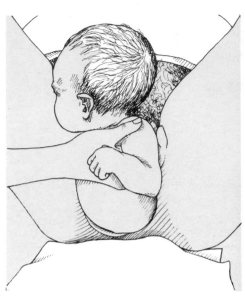

6 Supporting the baby's body, lift it up and over the mother's abdomen, and out of the birth canal. Avoid pulling on the cord.

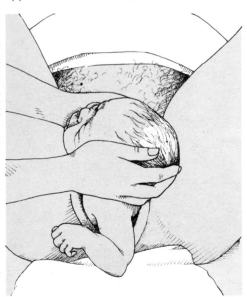

5 Lift upwards to allow the baby's lowermost shoulder to emerge from the birth canal.

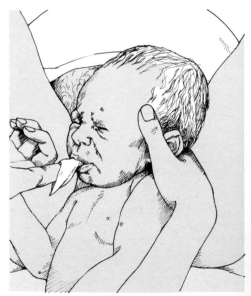

7 Lay the baby (still attached to the mother by the cord) between her legs. Clear out the baby's mouth with a swab, and he or she will normally begin to cry. Hold the baby very carefully because it will be very slippery.

8 Wrap the baby up in something soft and warm. Lay the baby on the side with the head low so that any fluid or mucus can drain from the mouth and nose

9 If the baby fails to respond, carry out the ABC of Resuscitation (see pp. 14–25).

DO NOT smack the baby.

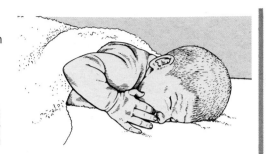

THE THIRD STAGE

At any time between 10 and 30 minutes after the birth of the baby, the *afterbirth* (placenta) should separate from the mother's womb. When it is about to be expelled, the mother will experience mild contractions. Encourage her to hold her breath and to push the afterbirth out. She will find this easiest if she is lying down with her knees up and apart. *Do not pull the afterbirth or cord while it is being expelled.*

There is no need to separate the afterbirth from the cord, this can safely be left until medical aid is available. Keep it intact, preferably in a polythene bag, as it will have to be examined for completeness when the mother reaches the hospital. Even a small piece left inside the mother can cause complications later.

When the afterbirth has been expelled, clean up the mother and lay a sanitary pad or clean towel over the vagina. Make her as comfortable as possible and encourage her to rest. A small amount of bleeding is normal. Severe bleeding rarely occurs, but, if this does happen, remember skilled help is on the way, so keep calm. Gently massage the mother's abdomen just below the navel to stimulate the uterus to contract. The uterus will harden as it contracts but continue massage until skilled help arrives.

To minimize shock, if it develops, treat the mother as on pp. 80 and 86.

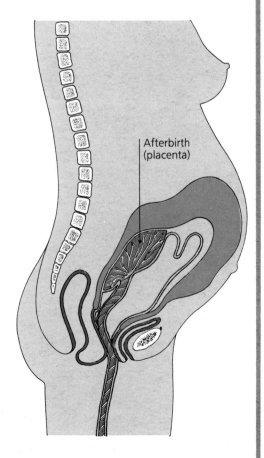

Afterbirth (placenta)

Third stage

DEALING WITH THE CORD

In most instances no harm will result if the umbilical cord is left attached to the baby until expert help arrives or the mother and baby reach hospital. If the cord is very short or removal to hospital will be delayed, it may be necessary to cut the cord. Wait until: after the afterbirth has been delivered; the cord has stopped pulsating; or until at least 10 minutes after the birth.

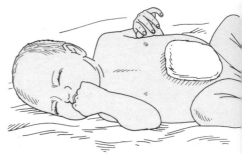

3 Place a sterile dressing over the cut end at the baby's abdomen.

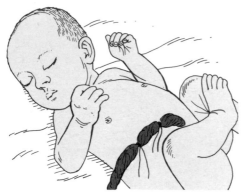

1 Using two of the prepared pieces of string (see p.209), tie the cord very firmly in two places: 15 cm (6 in) and 20 cm (8 in) from the baby's abdomen. If the piece of string nearest the baby is not tied very firmly the baby may bleed to death when the cord is cut.

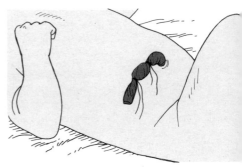

4 Ten minutes after cutting, inspect the cord to make sure there is no bleeding. Tie the remaining piece of string around the cord 10 cm (4 in) from the baby's abdomen.

5 Dress the cord again with another sterile dressing and secure it with a crepe or broad-fold bandage or by tying a folded napkin around the baby's abdomen.

IF there is no sterile dressing available, do not tie anything around the baby.

IF the cord has to be cut before the afterbirth has been expelled, cover the end of the umbilical cord attached to the afterbirth with a sterile dressing.

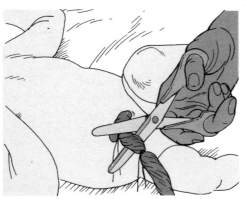

2 Cut the cord between the two ties using the sterilized scissors.

NOTE
Always keep the afterbirth so that it can be examined later.

APPENDICES

VOLUNTARY AID SOCIETY (V.A.S.) OBSERVATION CHART						

ASSESSMENT OF RESPONSE (mark with ✓ if yes)

NAME   **DATE**

TIME						
EYES OPEN	spontaneously					
	to speech					
	to pain					
	no response					
MOVEMENT	obeys command					
	to painful stimulus					
	no response					
SPEECH RESPONSE	normal					
	confused					
	inappropriate words					
	incomprehensible sounds					
	no response					
PULSE (beats per minute)	111–120					
	101–110					
	91–100					
	81–90					
	71–80					
	61–70					
	51–60					
RESPIRATION (breaths per minute)	41–50					
	31–40					
	21–30					
	11–20					
	1–10					

MANUAL ARTIFICIAL VENTILATION

There may be occasions in which Mouth-to-Mouth Ventilation cannot be used, and these might be:

■ If there are severe facial injuries involving both the casualty's mouth and nose.
■ If the casualty is trapped in a face-downwards position.
■ A case of poisoning (see p.152) where contamination around the casualty's mouth can affect the First Aider, e.g., corrosive substances, cyanide.

The Holger Nielsen Method is a manual ventilation technique but it is not as efficient as Mouth-to-Mouth. It cannot be used if there are serious injuries to the arms or the chest. It involves pushing on the chest from the back, to force air out of the lungs, then moving the casualty's arms upwards and outwards to expand the chest and produce inspiration.

As with normal resuscitation, a much lighter pressure and faster rate will be necessary when performing this method of resuscitation on children.

Checking for response

If resuscitation is successful, the casualty's colour will improve (see p.21). If no improvement is noticed after the first four ventilations, there may be an obstruction in the airway (see p.48), or the heart may have stopped beating (see p.17).

THE HOLGER NIELSEN METHOD

This is the next preferred method of Artificial Ventilation after Mouth-to-Mouth because it maintains the open airway while the casualty is in a face-downwards position. However, while the casualty is in this position you cannot perform External Chest Compression nor can you easily check for heartbeat or signs of response.

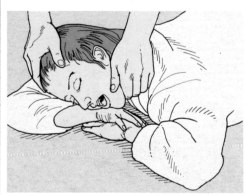 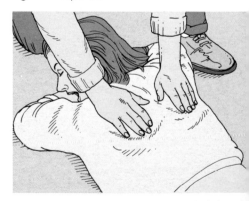

1 With the casualty face down on a hard flat surface, place her arms above her head and place her hands, one over the other, under her head. Turn her head to one side, with her cheek resting on her uppermost hand. Tilt her head back, and extend her jaw so that her airway is open.

2 Kneel on one knee at the casualty's head with your other foot at the point of her elbow. Place your hands on her back on top of the shoulder-blades; your thumbs should be along either side of the spine.

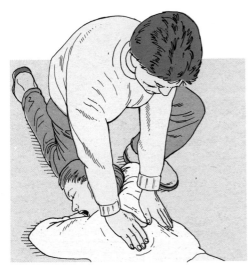

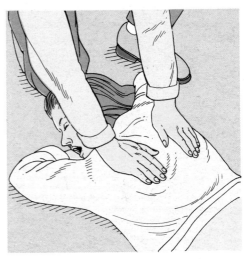

DO NOT overstretch.

3 Keep your elbows straight and rock forward until your arms are approximately vertical, exerting steady pressure for about two seconds. This makes the casualty exhale.

DO NOT apply too much pressure or you may damage her lungs and internal organs.

5 Lower the casualty's arms and slide your hands down on to her back again ready to repeat the cycle. Repeat the sequence rhythmically 12 times per minute; each cycle of expansion and compresssion should last for five seconds.

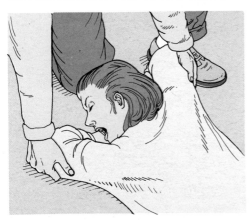

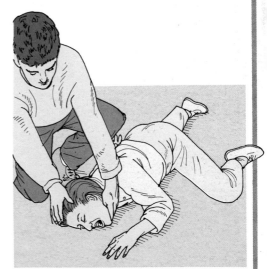

4 Rock backwards, sliding your hands upwards and outwards along the casualty's arms and grasp them just above her elbow. Raise her arms until resistance and tension are felt at the shoulder, about three seconds – this produces inspiration.

6 As soon as the casualty begins to breathe, place her in the Recovery Position (see p.24), if possible.

INDEX

ACKNOWLEDGMENTS

Editorial committee
Dr C.C. Molloy, St. John Ambulance Association
Dr J.W. Junor, St. Andrew's Ambulance Association
Brigadier D.D. O'Brien, British Red Cross Society

Consultants
St. John Ambulance Association: Dr P.A.B. Raffle, Dr J.H.E.
Baker, Mr P.S. London and Commander S.H. Glenny
St. Andrew's Ambulance Association: the late Dr H.R.F.
Macdonald and Mr G. Watt
British Red Cross Society: Mr E.A. Malkin, Miss M. Baker and
Mr J. Williams

Editor	Janice Lacock
Art editor	Tina Vaughan
Designers	Sarah Ponder, Tracy Timson
Managing editor	Daphne Razazan
Art director	Anne-Marie Bulat

Illustrators
Kuo Kang Chen, Coral Mula, Tony Randell, Mary Tomlin,
Adam Willis

Photography
All special photographs by Peter Chadwick; p.165 Rex Features

Typesetting
SX Composing Ltd.

Reproduction
A. Mondadori, Verona

Dorling Kindersley would like to thank:
Airedale Graphics, Richard and Hilary Bird, Ann Cannings,
Jim Cork, Mike Hearne, Martin Kirk, Jean and Richard Lacock,
Philip Lord, John Major, Trevor Norwood, St. John
Ambulance Association Branch London District, and all the
members of staff who modelled for the step-by-steps.